PRAISE FOR *WHY COPE WHEN YOU CAN HEAL?*

"COVID-19 has asked as much or more of the frontline healthcare worker as nothing before. We were not ready for this and we need help. Goulston and Hendel tell it like it is, providing clear, actionable, and deeply moving advice and tangible tools to ease the pain and prevent the worst. Healing is needed; solutions are at hand."

—RICHARD AFABLE, MD, MPH, PRESIDENT/BOARD CHAIR, BEWELL ORANGE COUNTY; RETIRED CEO, ST. JOSEPH HOAG HEALTH

"Thank you for writing this extremely important book. Burnout and mental health challenges were already a significant issue for healthcare clinicians before the COVID-19 pandemic. *Why Cope When You Can Heal?* heightens the reader's awareness of the additional trauma experienced now by the healthcare workforce and prepares them for the aftermath of COVID-19 and a potential parallel pandemic. The authors also acknowledge the tensions between health and the economy and individual freedom and the common good that are essential to manage in order to achieve a healthy public, a healthy workforce, and a strong economy. This is an important book for healthcare workers and leaders at all levels to read, so the trauma experienced by the healthcare workforce will not be ignored or dismissed, and those impacted will have the best opportunity to heal."

—TRACY CHRISTOPHERSON, PhD-c, MS, BAS, RRT AND MICHELLE TROSETH, MSN, RN, FNAP, FAAN, COFOUNDERS, MISSINGLOGIC; COHOSTS, *HEALTHCARE'S MISSINGLOGIC PODCAST*

"The authors have given us an important book to read and understand deeply in the midst of an unprecedented global pandemic and social upheaval. We have finally begun to understand the issues of burnout in healthcare professionals, and then we get hit with this challenge. Our ICU and ED professionals choose these areas of focus and have special aptitude and training in taking care of the most complex and precarious patients. After sharing with us the depth of emotion and pain that the professionals endure and deal with daily, the authors then provide strong insights into what the personal experiences and issues are and the extent of damage inflicted. But we are fortunate to then be shown with great clarity the diagnostic nuances, and then provided with proven therapeutics and interventions to provide these courageous and impacted colleagues with plans and pathways to not only survive and improve but even to heal. Thanks so much for writing this important book."

—JACK COCHRAN, RETIRED EXECUTIVE DIRECTOR (CEO), THE PERMANENTE FEDERATION OF KAISER PERMANENTE; AUTHOR, *HEALER, LEADER, PARTNER: OPTIMIZING PHYSICIAN LEADERSHIP TO TRANSFORM HEALTHCARE*

"The authors have achieved the rare feat of producing brilliant analysis, powerful and readable stories, and emotional engagement in the lives of those who work heroically to restore us and our loved ones to health. This book is a must-read blueprint for how to address an overlooked part of every crisis that strains our healthcare system."

—MICHAEL CRITELLI, RETIRED CHAIRMAN AND CEO, PITNEY BOWES; CEO, MOVEFLUX CORPORATION

"Healthcare providers always hold themselves accountable for the welfare of others but sometimes not for the welfare of themselves. This book provides great insights into emotional healing with the goal of not simply recovery but renewal of self and joy."

—CINDY EHNES, ESQ, PRINCIPAL, COPE HEALTH SOLUTIONS

"Why Cope When You Can Heal? is going to help lots of people. Thanks to Mark Goulston and Diana Hendel for explaining how PTSD affects healthcare providers and most importantly, how treatment can lead to recovery."

—DAVID FEINBERG, MD, VP, GOOGLE HEALTH; FORMER CEO, UCLA HEALTH; FORMER CEO, GEISINGER HEALTH SYSTEM

"As the CEO of an organization that touches almost half the healthcare delivered in the United States, we see the impact of burnout on providers and how COVID-19 has the potential to be the spark that ignites the catastrophic and permanent damage to the emotional well-being of our heroic frontline providers. *Why Cope When You Can Heal?* simply lays out a path for managing the trauma and is an important work in creating a foundation for healing with more than hope—concrete and practical pathways for recovery."

—HALEE FISCHER-WRIGHT, MD, MMM, FAAP, FACMPE, PRESIDENT AND CEO, MGMA; COAUTHOR, *TRIBAL LEADERSHIP* AND *BACK TO BALANCE*

"In order to care for others, healthcare providers need to maintain their own health and well-being. This book serves as a powerful blueprint for understanding, preventing, and healing from the traumatic stress unleashed by the COVID-19 pandemic. Even before this new challenge, the pressures on providers had produced crisis levels of burnout and suicide. In this moment, when it is easy to recognize that providers are heroes who return to the front lines every day, Goulston and Hendel offer a roadmap to empathy and recovery."

—STEVE A.N. GOLDSTEIN, MA, MD, PhD, FAAP, VICE CHANCELLOR HEALTH AFFAIRS, UNIVERSITY OF CALIFORNIA, IRVINE

"This quick and easy read will benefit many on the front lines of the COVID-19 pandemic and is an essential addition to any organization looking to help their teams thrive and build resilience in the midst of chronic stress and leadership burnout."

—MYRA GREGORIAN, CHIEF PEOPLE OFFICER, SEATTLE CHILDREN'S HOSPITAL

"This is the book we as clinicians need right now. Mark Goulston and Diana Hendel have articulated both the problem and solution for something we all realize: namely, that the pandemic is a human catastrophe, and that we need to help beyond just praise for the frontline heroes. The chapters on recovering from this trauma will save lives. I hope we all read it."

—STEPHEN K. KLASKO, MD, MBA, PRESIDENT AND CEO, THOMAS JEFFERSON UNIVERSITY AND JEFFERSON HEALTH; DISTINGUISHED FELLOW, WORLD ECONOMIC FORUM; AUTHOR, *UNHEALTHCARE: A MANIFESTO FOR HEALTH ASSURANCE*

"This book captures the urgency, humanity, passion, and utter devastation of this moment better than anything I've read. And yet, the book is hopeful, pointing to proven strategies that can heal our caregivers and our country and our world."

—DAVE LOGAN, PhD, CEO, CALIFORNIA MEDICAL ASSOCIATION (CMA) WELLNESS; *NEW YORK TIMES* BESTSELLING COAUTHOR OF *TRIBAL LEADERSHIP* AND *THE THREE LAWS OF PERFORMANCE*; FACULTY MEMBER, USC MARSHALL SCHOOL OF BUSINESS; COFOUNDER, CULTURESYNC

"A must-read for every healthcare provider or leader. It not only describes what we on the front lines have been faced with during these chaotic and unprecedented times but, even more importantly, it is filled with hope, inspiration, and lots of practical, evidence-based techniques and treatments for managing traumatic stress."

—JAGAT NARULA, MD, PhD, MAAC, CHIEF, DIVISION OF CARDIOLOGY, MOUNT SINAI MORNINGSIDE HOSPITAL

"Even prior to COVID-19, physician burnout was a national epidemic, with the highest suicide rate of any profession in the United States. COVID-19 brandished more stress and trauma on physicians, as well as all healthcare workers involved on the front lines of battling this pandemic. This book uniquely captures the raw emotions involved in this moment and offers hope, empathy, inspiration, and constructive solutions on how to heal and not just manage the emotional pain."

—SION ROY, MD, FACC, IMMEDIATE PAST PRESIDENT, LA COUNTY MEDICAL ASSOCIATION; TRUSTEE, SANTA MONICA COLLEGE

"Everyone knows healthcare workers are tough and resilient, but this pandemic has pushed most of us to the edge. Every nurse—in fact, everyone in healthcare—will benefit from the insights, tools, and support offered in this timely and easy-to-read guidebook."

—LISA SAUNIER, RN

"With insight and empathy, *Why Cope When You Can Heal?* opens the door and shows us a pathway toward much-needed healing. I hope that all organizations add this vital resource to their toolkits of support and guidance for all their employees who have served so well during this horrific time."

—NANCY SCHUTTENHELM, RN

"As a healthcare leader responsible for an organization of more than eighteen thousand healthcare providers and staff members, I care deeply about the emotional well-being of our team. This book is an essential resource for frontline providers and leaders alike, and is a terrific supplement to the programs and services we've implemented to help employees navigate the enormous stress of the COVID-19 pandemic."

—CHRIS D. VAN GORDER, FACHE, PRESIDENT/CEO
SCRIPPS HEALTH; AUTHOR, *THE FRONT-LINE LEADER*

"*Why Cope When You Can Heal?* will be a great resource for healthcare workers by providing a roadmap for continued good health. These are unprecedented times for all of our frontline healthcare personnel. A book like this is a great starting point to support our frontline staff and provide critical information for maintaining good mental health."

—MIKE WALL, FORMER PRESIDENT AND CEO, ST. JOHN'S
HOSPITAL IN SANTA MONICA, ANTELOPE VALLEY HOSPITAL,
NORTHRIDGE HOSPITAL, JOHN MUIR HEALTH SYSTEM

WHY COPE WHEN YOU CAN HEAL?

WHY COPE WHEN YOU CAN HEAL?

*How Healthcare Heroes of COVID-19
Can Recover from PTSD*

MARK GOULSTON, MD

DIANA HENDEL, PharmD

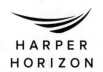

HARPER
HORIZON

Published by Harper Horizon, an imprint of HarperCollins Focus LLC.

Any internet addresses, phone numbers, or company or product information printed in this book are offered as a resource and are not intended in any way to be or to imply an endorsement by Harper Horizon, nor does Harper Horizon vouch for the existence, content, or services of these sites, phone numbers, companies, or products beyond the life of this book.

This book is designed to give information on various medical conditions, treatments, and procedures for your personal knowledge and to help you be a more informed consumer of medical and health services. It is not intended to be complete or exhaustive, nor is it a substitute for the advice of your physician. You should seek medical care promptly for any specific medical condition or problem you may have.

All efforts have been made to ensure the accuracy of the information contained in this book as of the date published. The authors and the publisher expressly disclaim responsibility for any adverse effects arising from the use or application of the information contained herein.

ISBN 978-0-7852-4476-9 (eBook)
ISBN 978-0-7852-4462-2 (TP)

Library of Congress Cataloging-in-Publication Data

Library of Congress Control Number: 2020945564

Printed in the United States of America
20 21 22 23   LSC   10 9 8 7 6 5 4 3 2 1

Dedicated to all healthcare providers, first responders, and essential workers, who daily put their lives at risk to keep the rest of the world safe.

CONTENTS

FOREWORD

When I was asked to write the foreword to Mark Goulston and Diana Hendel's *Why Cope When You Can Heal?* I was very excited, for many reasons. I still am. First of all, doctors, nurses, and other healthcare professionals are battered and bruised right now. They desperately need a way to process the extreme COVID-related trauma they are experiencing. The fact that leaders can hand them this book, with all of its powerful tools and tactics for healing, is a real gift.

But also, I am excited because I feel the subject of this book shows how far we have come as an industry.

Almost twenty years ago I wrote a book called *Hardwiring Excellence*. I'm grateful to say that since then it has sold more than a million and a half copies and is a staple in healthcare libraries. But at the time, nobody wanted to publish it. Why? Because it was considered "too soft." It was one of the first healthcare books that talked about employee engagement, its connection to the patient experience, and the fact that both are linked to clinical outcomes.

Healthcare has always been a complex industry. That was certainly true back when I wrote *Hardwiring Excellence*. Leaders were under huge pressure and struggling with complicated issues like payer mix, patient access, and rapidly rising costs. They were pulled in many different directions. And while they cared deeply about employees and patients (just as much as they do now), there were a lot of distractions.

With everything competing for their attention, it's understandable that employee engagement and patient experience weren't always top of mind.

Of course, once leaders realized the importance of these so-called soft skills and attitudes, they quickly refocused. I am happy to say that over the past couple of decades, the healthcare industry has made huge strides in these areas. Patient experience is now one of the most important metrics inside hospitals. And good leaders are realizing that employee engagement is key to clinical outcomes. In short, we now realize that passion, purpose, and a sense of worthwhile work is really what drives results and organization performance.

Even now, though, leaders can sometimes get pulled away from focusing on the soft stuff. In times of great crisis—like in the midst of a pandemic—it's not always easy to keep employee engagement and employees' emotional well-being front and center. But especially right now, we can't afford *not* to. It's the soft stuff that makes the hard stuff, like clinical outcomes and patient safety, work. Right now, employees may need the soft stuff just to get through another day.

Stephen Covey talks about the emotional bank account. He talks about it in terms of building trust with employees. I've always seen that bank account as the reservoir that feeds passion, purpose, and desire to make a difference. In healthcare we're lucky because we are in an industry where employees show up with a fully loaded emotional bank account. They see their work as a calling. I love to speak to a graduating class of nurses. These are some of the most engaged and excited people ever. They can't wait to start their journey. Over time, though, the nature of that work can drain the emotional bank account (not only for nurses but for all healthcare workers). It's up to leaders to make regular deposits to counteract the withdrawals.

That's what *Why Cope When You Can Heal?* helps us accomplish. And I think it serves many other purposes as well.

This book is a great reminder about the critical importance of self-care. As a profession, we focus on caring for others. We are truly passionate about that. But too often doctors, nurses, and other front-line workers don't take the time to care for themselves. When we don't practice self-care, we're focusing only on one prong of a two-pronged job. We've all heard the analogy about putting on our oxygen mask first. Healthcare professionals have the responsibility to stay mentally and emotionally well, so they'll have the inner resources to help patients heal.

It's up to leaders to teach employees to practice and prioritize that self-care. Left to their own devices, many employees will not do so. As Mark and Diana point out in *Why Cope When You Can Heal?*, healthcare workers tend to ignore their emotional wounds and soldier on. At times this may be a result of what the authors call healthcare's "just get over it" culture. But I also believe people keep on keeping on simply because they care so much. That's how mission-driven these people are. Part of the leader's role is to gently intervene where needed.

The book also shines a light on the importance of leader training. A huge part of the leader's role is giving people the tools they need to do the job. I'm not talking about personal protective equipment (PPE) here. I'm talking about leaders knowing *how* to help employees prevent and heal from post-traumatic stress disorder (PTSD). This kind of training may not have seemed so urgent in the past, but COVID-19 has brought it to the forefront. Training needs to evolve with changing circumstances.

Here's another reason that leaders need specialized training in the COVID-19 (and hopefully very soon, the *post*-COVID) era. Mark and Diana talk about the stigma around PTSD and other mental illnesses. Since leadership sets the tone for the hospital, it's important to ensure leaders get some training around this issue as well. When leaders are purposeful about breaking down the PTSD stigma, others will follow their lead.

Why Cope When You Can Heal? reminds us that we need a refocus on leadership fundamentals. Over the years we've found some tactics that work well for keeping employees engaged and connected to the larger sense of purpose that keeps them going: good performance management practices, leader rounding on employees, thank-you notes and other forms of reward and recognition, and so forth. Yet even organizations that do an effective job of hardwiring such tactics can drift away from them. In times of crisis we must bring ourselves back to these fundamentals. We need their good results, and the structure they provide, more than ever.

Take rounding, for instance. In terms of engagement tactics, this one is a powerhouse. Essentially, leaders put a system in place to make sure they meet regularly with each direct report. The idea is to ask a series of questions aimed at getting to know people and making sure they have what they need to do their best work. In the best of times, rounding is a tool for creating a great employee experience. In the worst of times, it's a lifeline for making a deep human connection, reducing uncertainty (and anxiety), and ensuring that employees are truly "okay."

In chapter 7, Diana writes about communication. She notes that even if we think we're communicating well, in times of crisis we almost certainly need to do even more. I've seen the truth of this over the years. When people hear nothing, they assume the worst. The more you check in, the less anxious they'll be. Rounding is a good tool for keeping people informed, but also be sure to share information in other ways. Employee forums. Hospital message boards. Emails. Videos. If it's worth saying, you can't say it too often.

I'm not just talking about sharing facts and answering questions. That type of communication matters, too, but connecting on an emotional level is even more vital. I've always been a fan of good storytelling. Why? Because stories connect to the heartstrings. They make things real for the listener. When we tell stories about that doctor or nurse who saved a life or made a profound impact, what people hear is "my work makes a real difference." Stories are great teaching tools. When we connect a story to a behavior, we inspire employees to do more of that behavior.

Stories also build community. They help staff members to see that, however deeply they are struggling, they're not alone. I feel one of the most important things leaders can do is give people space and time and attention to tell their COVID-19 stories. People want to be heard. Sharing their stories helps them process their anxiety, grief, and other strong emotions.

I'd like to share one more reason why I am grateful to be a part of this book. It's a good reminder that healthcare is an industry of heroes. This has always been true. I have known and worked with many of these heroes over the years. But reading about the heart-wrenching experiences frontline healthcare workers are facing right now is truly humbling. It reminds us of how passionate, dedicated, and courageous this profession truly is.

If our doctors, nurses, and other healthcare heroes can get through COVID-19, they can do anything. I know that they will. And we have a sacred trust to help them not just get through it but go on to thrive on the other side. We owe it to them to give them the tools and support they need to heal from the trauma they have faced and continue to face every day. We owe it to the patients we serve. And we owe it to the future of our industry, our nation, and our world.

QUINT STUDER, FOUNDER OF THE STUDER GROUP

WHY READ THIS BOOK?

If you've picked up this book, you are likely serving on the healthcare front lines of the COVID-19 pandemic, are directly supporting or leading those who do, or are the friend or family member of someone who is. You may be struggling and seeking help for yourself, for a coworker, or for others you know who have been directly impacted.

Healthcare is a challenging industry during the best of times. It demands fast thinking, steadiness under pressure, tenacity, and a passion for helping others. Healthcare workers have these qualities in abundance, and during normal times, while your job can sometimes be difficult, you are confident that you can handle inevitable challenges and feel good about your work.

But this pandemic is anything but normal. During COVID-19 you have likely faced a massive upheaval in your work life and your personal life. For some of you, your safety and the safety of your loved ones is compromised each time you go to work. And with the massive death toll associated with this coronavirus, your work life is punctuated by tragedy and death at every turn. You may even feel guilt or responsibility for some of these losses. It would not be surprising if you were struggling with all of this. COVID-19 takes a serious toll on the front lines.

Sadly, COVID-related trauma is real and serious. Many healthcare workers are at risk for developing Post-Traumatic Stress Disorder

(PTSD) due to the traumatic stress of working the front lines of the pandemic. We've seen this happen with SARS (severe acute respiratory syndrome) and Ebola in the past, and early research shows that some frontline workers are already experiencing PTSD symptoms. Traumatic stress can be debilitating and horrific, and this is the last thing you need when you are duty bound by your work.

But even if you are experiencing traumatic stress, there is so much hope for a healthy and bright future to look forward to and live into. You can heal and gain new levels of strength to sustain you during the remainder of this pandemic and beyond. This book is an alternative to suffering in silence. It offers healthcare workers clarity, healing, and hope.

We guide you through the traumatizing factors impacting your life in today's "new normal" circumstances. This step is valuable because when you name the (many) elements that are causing your pain, you begin to process or "tame" them. Further, reading firsthand experiences of other healthcare professionals validates your own feelings and reminds you that you are not going through this alone. As you read these, keep in mind that these accounts may be triggering. So be kind and gentle with yourself, and if you need additional support don't hesitate to reach out to friends, family, or a mental health professional.

Why Cope When You Can Heal? shares therapeutic approaches that are currently used to effectively treat traumatic stress and PTSD—including a new approach called Surgical Empathy—and introduces powerful exercises to help you move through the trauma and further your healing. While this book is not intended to provide comprehensive treatment for PTSD, or to completely resolve your trauma-related symptoms, it provides a starting point for healing and offers many resources to support you along the way.

If you're a leader you, too, will benefit from this book. In it are guidelines for effective communication and listening, and suggestions for trauma-informed support services. When empathetic and supportive leaders ensure the safety of workers, decrease uncertainty, and unify the workforce, the damaging effects of traumatic stress on individuals can be reduced. Thus morale improves, collaboration increases, and turnover is minimized, all of which benefit the organization as a whole—and the patients and community it serves.

There's no doubt that traumatic stress is a formidable foe, but there is relief from your suffering. In this book we offer you the possibility of healing. And with healing comes hope.

CHAPTER 1

A PERFECT STORM
FOR TRAUMA

This is the story of a worldwide pandemic and how its grim realities—along with many devastating political and cultural facets of our national response—have coalesced in a way that has deeply traumatized US healthcare professionals. To borrow a familiar analogy, these workers have been forced to cope with a perfect storm of factors that have overwhelmed and battered their psyches to an unprecedented degree.

As we write these words in the midsummer of 2020, the COVID-19 pandemic continues to surge, and hundreds of thousands of people have died worldwide. With the caveat that the pandemic is an evolving situation, let's briefly review what has transpired. We think readers will agree: this global crisis, which has altered virtually everything about our world, has unfolded at shocking speed.

IT ALL HAPPENED SO QUICKLY

In late December 2019 reports began circulating that a pneumonia-like virus was making people sick in Wuhan, China. Symptoms included a cough, fever, shortness of breath or difficulty breathing, and a loss of smell and/or taste.

On January 11, 2020, the first known death resulting from an illness caused by the 2019 novel coronavirus was reported by the Chinese media.[1]

Over the following days, the first cases outside of mainland China began to crop up. Confirmed cases occurred in Japan, South Korea, Thailand, and the US.

Because we live in an age where international travel is the norm, global spread may have been inevitable. People contracted the highly contagious virus and went about their daily lives. As they came into contact with others, they unknowingly passed it on to them, and those people infected still others.

On January 30, with nearly ten thousand reported cases worldwide, the World Health Organization (WHO) declared the unfolding situation a pandemic. The next day the Trump administration declared a public health emergency in the US and set quarantines for Americans who had recently traveled to certain parts of China. The pandemic had hit home—and it hit hard.

In February people in the US started dying of the virus. Within weeks those first few deaths would become an avalanche, and on March 13 President Trump declared a national emergency and Congress approved funding of up to $50 billion for states and territories to combat the spreading coronavirus.[2]

By March 26 the US had the highest number of COVID-19 cases in the world, with at least 81,321 infections and over 1,000 deaths.[3] Nationwide, massive efforts to "flatten the curve" and keep hospitals from being overrun were already well underway. For the rest of our lives, we will surely remember these days. Nonessential businesses closed and office workers set up shop at home. Education went online. Sports seasons were cancelled. Churches were closed. Every aspect of our lives changed drastically . . . and it happened shockingly fast.

People were initially asked to stay home if possible and, when they did go out, to stay six feet apart and wear face coverings. But great controversy surrounded these recommendations and the orders to stay at home. Some people focused on saving the US economy and others insisted that no price was too high to pay for saving human lives. With financial pressure and hardship mounting, locked-down states began to reopen in phases over the spring and early summer. There was little consistency from state to state, and within weeks new surges in infection rates and deaths resulted.

At the time of this writing, the ideological battle between those who want to save the economy by reopening the country and those who seek to maximize the preservation of life at all costs continues—and as COVID-19 surges across the country, many hotspots are debating closing down again. There is no end in sight. The uncertainty about the future is itself a traumatizing factor.

HEALTHCARE WORKERS FACE WAR-TIME CONDITIONS

Besides having to process the speed and intensity with which "normal" life has been altered—and in many cases dealing with grief and worry over loved ones who've been infected with this novel coronavirus—healthcare professionals have faced incredible hardship in their work. They've seen and done things that have scarred them for life. In many ways their working environment became a war zone almost overnight.

At the beginning doctors, nurses, paramedics, and other health-care workers braced for a massive influx of sick patients. Hospital leaders launched government-recommended, stringent infection-control protocols as they went into "surge" mode, setting up triage tents and dedicating floors and wings for coronavirus patients. And they prepared for the grim likelihood that a shortage of beds and

ICU equipment would force them to make impossible life-and-death decisions.

The war-time nature of the pandemic became clear when hospitals had to move patients from place to place, set up special COVID units, and in some cases take even more extreme measures to manage the load.

For example, King County in Washington State set up a two-hundred-bed field hospital on a nearby soccer field, and an army field hospital went up at CenturyLink Field, home of the Seattle Seahawks, to help relieve medical centers swamped by coronavirus.[4]

In New York City—which became the first US epicenter of the pandemic with a horrifically high death rate occurring in a compressed time period—refrigerated trucks lined the streets outside of hospitals, set up as temporary morgues. The bodies of COVID-19 victims that went unclaimed after a period of time were buried in mass graves on New York's Hart Island.[5]

Through it all, while healthcare providers were busy caring for their patients, they were getting infected themselves (considering the shortage of personal protective equipment [PPE] they've had to deal with, this is no surprise). As of June 3, 2020, the coronavirus had infected at least 450,000 healthcare workers worldwide, according to a report issued by an international nursing federation.[6]

Of the healthcare workers infected, nearly six hundred were reported dead by early June, including doctors, nurses, and paramedics, along with support staff such as administrators, nursing home workers, and hospital janitors.[7]

The horrific realities of working in healthcare during a pandemic cannot be understated. Healthcare staffers must work exhausting hours and isolate from their families for weeks on end. They must comfort patients who die alone with no soothing human touch, and comfort family members who must say goodbye via video screen (if at all). This takes a toll.

THEY FACE A DISTRESSING LACK OF SUPPORT

It would be bad enough to work on the front lines of a pandemic in a strong healthcare system that's part of a stable, supportive, and united country. From supply-chain issues, to clear and concise guidelines, to messaging and instructions to the public, there has been a lack of a cohesive plan for the country. Unfortunately, healthcare leaders and workers must do their incredibly difficult jobs inside a healthcare system that is often disjointed and fragmented and part of a deeply divided nation wracked by strife.

Many decry the dilution of the influence of organizations like the CDC and WHO, thought leaders the healthcare industry has long looked to for regulation and support. For healthcare leaders and workers, the lack of a cohesive national plan, along with sensing that the expertise and guidance of scientists are being ignored or minimized, is extremely troubling (remember, these are people who've been steeped in the importance of science and evidence).

Further, it is difficult for healthcare workers to consistently instill hope, confidence, and reassurance in their patients, because of the inconsistent and contradictory messages in the media and from national figureheads. Psychologically managing these inconsistencies only adds to their stress.

One of the most personal impacts of America's lack of pandemic readiness has been equipment shortages like virus tests, ventilators, and PPE. It's not easy to work every day knowing you lack the necessities to keep patients safe. And when you must resort to baking single-use masks in the oven so you can reuse them the next day, or wearing a garbage bag as a gown, you feel devalued and incredibly vulnerable.

Meanwhile, healthcare organizations' budgets are imperiled, leading to massive job loss and job insecurity across the industry. As the nation went into lockdown and elective procedures were cancelled, more than a million healthcare workers were furloughed and laid off.

Many others had their salaries cut. Survivors of initial job losses found themselves living in fear that they were next.

Living and working in these horrific conditions—combined with the intensity, duration, and open-endedness of this pandemic—is enough to break anyone. None of us have seen anything like this before. All these factors are culminating in a perfect storm that has the potential to push healthcare workers into PTSD.

THE JUST-GET-OVER-IT CULTURE MAKES A BAD SITUATION WORSE

And there's one other huge factor that plays into all of this: America's just-get-over-it culture. This has created a double whammy for healthcare providers in terms of trauma. The big push to quickly reopen the country is a reflection of this culture. And as more and more businesses reopened (too soon, in the eyes of many experts), the virus surged in many places. As a result, healthcare workers have gotten little relief from their workload and its heavy psychological toll. There has been no time to process emotions, a fact that will surely lead many to experience PTSD down the road.

But also—and this is the second part of the double whammy—healthcare has its own version of the just-get-over-it culture. In some organizations workers are expected to buck up, figure it out, get it done with the equipment they have, and move on to the next patient. Trying to navigate a pandemic in such a culture (where burnout is already rife) is pushing workers to the breaking point.

In chapter 2 we will explore firsthand accounts of the traumatic experiences that many of your colleagues in the industry have lived through. You will have a chance to recognize, name, and claim feelings you yourself are likely struggling with as the virus rages on.

Reading these accounts will empower you to give names to the anxiety, fear, stress, hopelessness, and helplessness you are dealing with. They will validate your feelings as perfectly normal—especially in these far-from-normal circumstances. They will also give you comfort in knowing you are not alone in these feelings. Finally, the accounts will help you process and heal from the trauma that stems from these kinds of experiences.

The bottom line is this: we all have to face the realities of the COVID-19 pandemic, and healthcare workers have a close-up view. All you can do is move through it one day at a time. What you don't have to do is resign yourself to the long-term aftereffects of trauma. There is a path to recovery from traumatic stress and PTSD. Why merely cope when you can heal?

CHAPTER 2

THE FRONTLINE EXPERIENCE:

A Look at the Tragedies and Traumas Surrounding the Pandemic

On May 16, 2020, the *New York Times* reported that a young anonymous nurse was the only person allowed in the hospital room of a seventy-five-year-old man dying from COVID-19. The nurse dimmed the lights and played soft music, made him as comfortable as she could, and held his hand. Close to the end of his life, she held up an iPad so he could see and hear a grief-stricken relative who was just outside in the hospital corridor. After the patient died, the nurse went to a secluded hallway and wept.[1]

This is only one story, but it reflects the experiences of many healthcare workers in the pandemic. Frontline healthcare providers across the nation are fighting the good fight for patients. They are risking their lives to save others. They are standing vigil as patients die. They are comforting devastated family members. Healthcare workers are no doubt heroes, but they are also human. And their heroic service comes at a high cost as they take on the heartbreak and tragedy of this deadly virus.

As healthcare workers face the pandemic, their personal and professional worlds collide. On the work front they are battling an invisible enemy that no one yet knows how to defeat. Their days are spent trying to treat a massive influx of patients—many of whom die horrible deaths before their very eyes. This takes a tremendous personal toll; not only do healthcare providers feel helpless to save many of their patients but they cannot even allow patients' loved ones to provide final moments of comfort. It is the nurses, the CNAs, the doctors, and the other staff who take up the mantle of helping strangers transition into death. The sheer volume of these relentless experiences only adds to their emotional burden and grief.

Add to this the risk of infection that every healthcare worker fears. Each moment spent in the room with a COVID-19 patient is a risk to their own health. Each intubation process is a chance of exposure. And with the severely limited supplies of PPE that healthcare facilities have faced, workers must resort to hoarding and reusing masks and other protective gear.

Healthcare workers also risk exposing their partners, their children, and their aging parents and other family members to the virus, not to mention their entire communities. They must be supremely vigilant to avoid bringing the virus home, and many have chosen to isolate themselves or their family members to decrease the chances of a transmission.

And then there's the issue of shortages in medical equipment. In the early months hospitals had to fight for ventilators and testing was at times severely limited. Adding insult to injury, doctors nationwide have looked on with disbelief and anger as some citizens shirk social distancing guidelines or choose not to wear masks when social distancing is impossible.

Another reason the pandemic is so traumatizing is because it is so open-ended. With a vaccine at least a year away from the onset of the pandemic, healthcare providers wonder how long they can keep up this pace.

Now we will look into factors that have caused healthcare workers—including you—so much pain. You may have experienced some or even all of these firsthand. But even if you have not, reading the visceral accounts below might provide you with valuable "aha" moments when someone in your industry accurately describes the emotions or feelings you've been trying to pinpoint or put into words.

Let's be clear: The events, feelings, and fears featured below may be overwhelming and traumatizing to the reader, especially when read all at once. But as you read, remember that the goal is to identify and acknowledge the pain that you and others in your industry are facing right now—not to dwell in it or feel hopeless. When you begin healing (hopefully in the very near future!), chances are these painful memories and feelings surrounding the pandemic will not have the same impact on you that they do today.

And by the way, it's not just doctors and nurses whose lives have been greatly impacted by COVID-19. All healthcare personnel working on the front lines have been touched by the traumatizing factors that this book focuses on. This group includes respiratory care practitioners, pharmacists, lab technicians, physician assistants, medical assistants, phlebotomists, admitting personnel, custodial staff, certified nursing assistants, home healthcare providers, emergency medical technicians, physical therapists, occupational therapy aides, speech-language pathologists, healthcare leaders, and so many more.

What follows are actual accounts from healthcare professionals of situations, in some cases horrific situations, that they've experienced during this pandemic. Our intention is neither to sensationalize COVID-19 events nor trigger upset in the readers we aim to help. Rather, we seek to document these occurrences, because *they happened* and we don't want them to be lost in the rush to put COVID-19 behind us once effective vaccines and treatments are developed.

We are determined that, as the world rushes to move past this tragedy, the heroes of COVID-19 who continue to struggle psychologically will not be forgotten or disregarded as were many of the heroes from other wars. And make no mistake about it: we are in a war. To that end we are unwavering in our commitment to prevent COVID-19 heroes with PTSD from following in the tragic footsteps of the veterans who die by suicide each day.

If you are a frontline healthcare worker, it may be difficult to be reminded of these experiences. But it is important to understand the reasons upon reasons that COVID-19 is such a traumatizing crisis for you and your colleagues. By breaking down the traumatic factors you have been living and working with since the beginning of the pandemic, you can hopefully give names to some of the feelings you may be struggling to identify and begin to process each wound. Remember, if you can name it you can tame it.

That said, take this section slowly and be gentle with yourself as you read. It is meant to comfort you by showing you that you are not alone. It is not meant to agitate you. If at any point you feel it is too intense or uncomfortable to continue reading, stop and take a break. You may want to bring some of these topics into your next therapy session. Or you might reach out to a work colleague to share how you are feeling. And if you need urgent help, call 911 immediately. Other support is also available by phone, text, or in person.[2]

Here is a look at what healthcare workers are experiencing due to COVID-19:

THEY ARE ROCKED BY FEAR OF THE UNKNOWN

The coronavirus is an invisible enemy if ever there was one. It kills some and spares others. It can go undetected in an asymptomatic person for weeks or indefinitely.[3]

It spreads through the air, and aerosolized viral particles can stay airborne for hours.[4] No one is entirely sure how to prevent the virus's spread. Any one of the above realities is enough to traumatize the healthcare workers charged with treating the sick. Then consider that no one knows exactly how to treat the virus and that we are a long time from a vaccine. The uncertainties stack up. *How long will this go on? Will there be enough supplies? Will there ever be a vaccine?*

THEY FACE MASSIVE AMOUNTS OF ILLNESS AND DEATH WHILE PUTTING ON A BRAVE FACE

One can face only so much death before it takes a toll. Normally healthcare workers are expected to stoically accept death and keep on working. Nonetheless, they feel deep grief and sorrow when a patient dies. What's different about COVID-19 is being bombarded by death—so much that their COVID units (and sometimes the adjacent hallways) are overflowing with dying patients and hospital hallways are lined with body bags.[5]

Healthcare workers have no choice but to deal with the onslaught and keep fighting to do what they can.

In April, Jason Hill, who works in Manhattan at two New York-Presbyterian hospitals wrote,

> My colleagues are tired. The patients keep coming. The ER is wall-to-wall misery and mayhem. Only five people died on me today.

Only five. But everyone there is dying to varying degrees and at various rates. The ER is a cross section of the disease: The well who will stay well. The well who will come back much worse. The sick who are stable. The sick who are crashing. It's all around us. It keeps coming in through the front door. It keeps coming in through the ambulance bay. And my colleagues are tired. We give oxygen. Everyone staying gets oxygen. Needs oxygen. We try antibiotics. We try antivirals. We try hydroxychloroquine. This week we use steroids. This week we limit IV fluids. This week we give blood thinners. Does anything work? Are we saving anyone, or just supporting them as they go along a path predetermined by the virus coursing through their insides? Is the inevitable inevitable? Some days, we just feel like spectators, front-row observers going through the necessary scenes of a play whose final act has already been written. So much death. So much dying. And my colleagues are tired. We're all tired.[6]

THEY ARE RUNNING ON FUMES (BUT THEY CAN'T STOP TO REST, RECOVER, OR PROCESS)

It's worth repeating: healthcare workers are tired. They work long shifts that they compare to living nightmares. They post photos of their exhausted faces marked by red and purple bruises caused by their PPE. They work twenty-four-hour shifts so they can make fewer trips home and lower the risk of passing the virus on to family members and other citizens. But what's more, they don't have time to hit pause—the need for healthcare workers is too great. This means they don't have the time or ability to pause, reflect, and process the crisis that continues grinding away at them. And so they carry on for as long as they are able. "I honestly have no idea how I feel," said Matthew Bai, a physician at Mount Sinai Hospital in Manhattan. "I go to work, and at the end of the day, I go to sleep. I have no time to digest any of this."[7]

THEY ARE RACKED BY ANXIETY, DEPRESSION, GRIEF, AND MORE

As doctors witness the ongoing horror of COVID-19, their levels of anxiety and depression (along with fear and grief) have risen to an all-time high. "I'm dealing with a lot of anxiety," said Kimberley Brown, an emergency room physician serving in northern Mississippi. "Right now, I feel really alone because very few people can kind of understand where my head is at. I'm just worried about getting sick. I'm worried about people around me getting sick. And my mind keeps going back to my colleagues in other parts of the country who are currently hospitalized in the ICU from COVID. And it scares me 'cause, I mean, I'm not that much younger than them."[8]

"What is it like being a nurse in a pandemic?" wrote registered nurse Emily Pierskalla in a blog post titled "I Want My Death to Make You Angry." "Every day I bounce through the stages of grief like a pinball. The ricochet and whiplash leaves my soul tired and bruised."[9] Doctors Arghavan Salles and Jessica Gold reported that "we have anger, sadness, fear, and anxiety, immense feelings that seem to come out of nowhere, like a tidal wave, and scare us. We choke them down to just do our jobs. Because that is what doctors are supposed to do."[10]

Some healthcare providers also describe tensions mounting at work. Brendan, a twenty-four-year-old paramedic firefighter who works forty-eight-hour shifts on the north side of St. Louis, told the *New York Times* that he goes for long stretches without eating, sleeping, or showering. "We are a lot quicker to be angry with each other," he said. "Any little thing sends us over the edge. But among the older guys in their late 30s and 40s, it's not OK to talk about things. So all anyone talks about is alcohol."[11]

The anxiety and depression don't just disappear once they leave work. Elizabeth Bonilla, a paramedic for the New York City Fire Department, told NPR that she has trouble sleeping in between her sixteen-hour shifts. Now she sleeps with the light on and plays gospel songs and yoga music. "It's hard for me to fall asleep in the dark because I get the image of that lady or that man who either passed away or who's suffering," Bonilla said. "I hear the cries. I hear the agony of people suffocating, trying to breathe."[12]

THEY EXPERIENCE INTENSE, OVERWHELMING, AND UNFORGETTABLE MOMENTS WITH PATIENTS AND PATIENTS' LOVED ONES

As frontline workers—doctors, nurses, CNAs, paramedics, firefighters, front-desk employees, and other essential healthcare workers—are facing the tidal wave of people sick and dying with COVID-19, they are witnesses and participants in the grueling and intense business of tending to the very sick and dying. They remember the anguish on patients' faces as they struggle to breathe. They make final phone calls or hold up tablets so family members can say goodbye to their loved ones, and they bear witness to the heartbreak, love, and grief. They remember watching patients slowly slip away. Every memory takes a toll.

Elizabeth Bonilla described responding to calls as "coming face to face with a monster that's overtaken a patient's body." She told NPR. com, "It's almost like the virus is talking to you. As soon as you see a patient, it's like, 'Oh, yeah, this person has the virus, . . . They're pale in the face. Some of them are blue in the lips, blue in the fingers, blue in their toes. They're panting like a dog."[13]

Prateek Harne, a resident physician in internal medicine at State University of New York (SUNY) Upstate Medical University, wrote on CNN.com,

My first encounter with a Covid-19 positive patient is something I will never forget. She had been admitted three days earlier, and I was asked to evaluate her, as her oxygen requirements had dramatically increased. As I stood in her room, my heart was racing. I didn't quite realize it in the moment, but I was scared.

With a distinct heaviness in her breath, she told me how nice everyone has been to her in the hospital. I thanked her. After examining her, I told her that we would need to intubate—insert a tube into her airway—for her to breathe better, and she replied by telling me she was very scared. I held her hand and told her it takes courage to do what she was doing. She asked me to call her husband, who was being quarantined at home after testing positive, and tell him that she loved him a lot. I did what she asked, and he asked me if I could tell her the same.

Four days later, she passed away due to severe respiratory failure, despite maximal medical supportive therapy. When I learned this, I went from being anxious to scared and then eventually subdued. I believe my anxiety came from three causes: The clinical unpredictability of the disease, its high transmissibility and, more importantly, not being able to alleviate my patient's distress.

Ever since then, every time I have entered a patient room with a potential Covid-19 infection I have felt scared—scared that I will infect other patients, my colleagues or my loved ones.[14]

Anne Cerniglia, an ICU nurse at Louisiana's Our Lady of the Lake Hospital, penned an article titled "What's It Like on the Front Lines? It's Hell."

I'm having to call a family on Zoom so they can say "goodbye" to their eldest sibling.

This is just the beginning of my shift, it's not even 8 a.m.

I gather up the phone numbers. We get everyone connected. We can't get the pastor connected. I get my gear on and go in the room with the tablet. I explain to the family, "We know it won't be much longer and we wanted to give you the opportunity to speak with your sibling. The blood pressure keeps getting lower and lower despite the three different types of medicines we have to make that pressure go up."

I let them know their family member was a fighter and they fought like hell for two weeks!

The family prays over the patient. They start singing a gospel song. My goggles are getting foggy and my mask is getting wet from my tears. How do you tell a family, "I'm sorry guys I can't continue to leave the tablet in the room for you to be with your sibling alone. I'm sorry I have to end this call because we are allotted 5 minutes and I've given y'all 15 minutes. I'm sorry I have to end this very last phone call ever with your sibling."

They understood. The call is over.[15]

THEY SUFFER MORAL INJURY

One of the hardest struggles healthcare providers face is the moral injury, the damage done to their conscience or moral compass when they are unable to prevent acts that transgress their deeply held moral beliefs, values, or ethics. Moral injury often describes the mental health toll on soldiers or those in the humanitarian field facing difficult or impossible situations and circumstances that are beyond their control.

Healthcare workers have made impossible life-or-death decisions. They have watched from behind goggles and face masks as patients slip away, unable to touch them or give them the comfort they deserve. They have grieved over patients who died alone because the patients dying outnumbered available staff.

"This is a disgusting kind of medicine that we are not used to," said Dr. Ninfa Mehta, medical director of the emergency department at SUNY Downstate Medical Center in Brooklyn, New York. "It's going to break people's hearts. Thinking that people are going to die alone, God, it's hard not to put yourself in the shoes of every patient you see."[16]

Ramona Moll, an ER nurse at the University of California, Davis Medical Center described feeling moral injury when she cannot touch or comfort her patients—and when they are unable to hear her over the whirr of the ventilators and fans. "You almost feel like a robot, because you can't communicate with them, you can't explain to them; the best you can do is, with your eyes, show compassion," she says.[17]

Derek Villareal has felt the impact as well. The ICU nurse at the Manhattan Veterans Affairs Hospital told NPR that he is haunted by the stream of desperate calls from patients' loved ones who aren't permitted to visit and knowing he has no time to comfort them. "We've been so inundated with phone calls, it's hard to talk about the death process with very concerned family members," Villareal said. "Again, these are things that really take you away from feeling like you were a good nurse that day."[18]

THEY ARE STRESSED AND WORRIED OVER PPE SHORTAGES

Without adequate PPE, the virus will spread among healthcare workers and the community. Massive nationwide shortages on PPE like gowns, gloves, N95 masks, and face shields have left healthcare providers terrified that they will have to work without sufficient coverage. And in many cases, those shortages have indeed occurred. Reports abound of frontline healthcare employees reusing PPE or being forced to get creative to find new (and questionable) ways to protect themselves from the virus. In March 2020 the hashtags #GetMePPE and #GetUsPPE were trending on social media outlets.[19]

Many workers have been forced to reuse their masks to make dwindling supplies last longer (something that never would have occurred prior to COVID-19). But now they keep their masks in Tupperware containers. They spray them with Lysol or alcohol in an attempt to sanitize them. They guard them like the precious resources they are.

Jason Hill described heating his mask in the oven to try to kill any virus present. He wrote,

> I'm baking a mask tonight. My single-use N95 has been on my face for days. The backs of my ears are raw from its straps rubbing, and my nostrils are filled with the scent of the fibers mixed with my coffee-flavored breath. My mask bakes and bakes in my oven, 70 degrees Celsius for 30 minutes every night, sterilizing it and killing any viral hitchhikers that attached themselves today. I wish I could do the same for someone's lungs. It comes out warm and toasty and clean. It comes out safe. I set it on the windowsill to cool, like an apple pie from easier days. Worst dessert ever.[20]

Some healthcare providers are taking matters into their own hands by crafting their own PPE out of other materials. They are making gowns out of garbage bags and some are even using plastic bags in place of face shields. And once they have their PPE securely in place, they don't want to remove it until absolutely necessary. Jaclyn O'Halloran wrote, "It is not uncommon for nurses to go all day without drinking water or eating because that would mean removing our protective gear."[21]

An article on Bloomberg.com reported the experiences of Marney Gruber, a physician who rotates through four New York City hospitals:

> She goes to work most days feeling vulnerable in her personal protective equipment. When she arrived for work at 10 p.m. Wednesday, she pulled on two pairs of gloves; a standard surgical mask tied over an N95 respirator mask; then a face shield and a scrub cap. For the next 10-and-a-half hours, she avoided the restroom: If she uses it, she's supposed to toss some of her one-time-use gear in the garbage. At the recommendation of hospital administrators, she's been using some of those supplies, like the N95, as long as a week, even though they are supposed to be discarded after seeing a single sick person.[22]

THEY FEEL HELPLESS

Healthcare workers struggle with the powerlessness of trying to help but often being unable to save patients, many of whom rapidly deteriorate. They feel as if they can't do enough for their patients due to a lack of protective gear or staffing shortages or simply not being able to save patients' lives. Elizabeth Bonilla described feeling helpless after seeing so many patients go into cardiac arrest. "You have just your little tools in your little bag," she said. "Most of our medications—I want to say all of our medications—don't even work on the patient."[23]

Jason Hill recounted that the only support he can provide is by offering patients a few creature comforts.

> I give out more juice and blankets than I ever have. In peacetime, the ER is busy, always busy—but most people are not dying. Very few are dying, and even fewer are acutely and actively dying. The scourge of COVID-19 has rewritten those rules. Everyone in the ER tonight is too sick to go home. Many are dying. Many will never

leave the hospital. Many will never have a meal or a juice box again. In peacetime, I often can't be bothered to bring someone juice. It's not a priority. Tonight, anyone asking gets juice. Even those not asking get juice. Often it's the only comfort I can provide—a small ease of suffering, a brief distraction from the fear. It may be the last juice they ever drink. Some nights, it's the best medicine I have.[24]

THEIR HIGHEST PERFORMERS ARE STILL NO MATCH FOR COVID-19

The healthcare industry attracts the very best and brightest, many of whom go on to do extraordinary things in their careers. These high performers are naturally resilient, skilled, tough, resourceful, and hard driving (or they never would have made it through the demands of medical school or met the high bar set in healthcare training). But even the toughest and most driven individuals are no match for something as destructive and beyond their control as COVID-19. The pandemic flooded them with overwhelming feelings of powerlessness, hopelessness, helplessness, and meaninglessness. And when high achievers who pride themselves on solving problems and making progress experience these things, they can buckle under pressure. Dr. Lorna Breen was one such individual.

Dr. Breen was a brilliant overachiever who lived her life with drive and certainty. She answered her life's calling to be a doctor by supervising the ER department at New York-Presbyterian Allen Hospital. But when COVID-19 sent her hospital reeling, Dr. Breen was overwhelmed like never before. After becoming infected with the novel coronavirus herself in March—and taking just a few days off of work to recover—she returned to work and struggled to catch up amid the chaotic scene. She reported to friends that this was the "hardest time of my life" and that "I'm drowning right now." Then she stopped responding to her friends altogether. Finally, on April 9, Dr. Breen reached out to her sister to ask for help. Despite worrying that her career would never recover, she checked herself into a psychiatric ward after suffering a breakdown. After eleven days she was discharged and went to stay with her mother. Though she initially seemed to be improving, she died by suicide on April 26.[25]

Dr. Breen was a giant in the healthcare industry, and even she collapsed under the hopelessness of the pandemic. Her story begs the question: If COVID-19 can bring down somebody like her, what can it do to the rest of the healthcare industry?

THEY FEEL DEEPLY RESPONSIBLE FOR THEIR PATIENTS' LIVES

Healthcare workers' sense of personal responsibility comes both from within (many answered a personal calling to save lives) and from outside pressures. During normal times it's common for them to second-guess the outcome when a patient who seemed to have no risk factors goes quickly south. But thanks to the unpredictable lethality of COVID-19, they are now hypersensitive of not assuming the worst-case outcome for every COVID-19 patient. And yes, they continue to be personally impacted by the losses for years. Despite the assumption that doctors and other care providers deal with death all the time, a tragic and unexpected death of a patient is typically a rare event that can haunt them for the rest of their lives.

THEY FEEL ISOLATED AND STIGMATIZED

Even with the nationwide push to celebrate healthcare providers, many feel completely alone, if not ostracized by their communities.

Some have described facing icy or hostile treatment in public or being shunned by neighbors. Some have stopped wearing scrubs in public because of the stigma of working among COVID-19 patients. On top of that, many are finding it hard to relate to friends, spouses, and family members, and only feel understood with coworkers who are experiencing the same things they are.

THEY ARE TERRIFIED OF CATCHING THE CORONAVIRUS (OR THEY'VE ALREADY CAUGHT IT)

Healthcare workers are among those most at risk of contracting the coronavirus, because they are constantly exposed to COVID-19 patients at work. They have seen firsthand what the virus can do and worry that they, too, will catch it. This adds another layer of fear to an already terrifying situation, especially with PPE in such short supply in many hospitals, urgent care centers, and nursing homes. In addition to constantly worrying about their exposure, healthcare workers second-guess every cough, headache, or sore throat. Healthcare workers are also talking with their spouses about worst-case scenarios. Many are getting their finances in order and updating their advanced directives.

And then there are the ones who contracted COVID-19 and suffered not only from the debilitating symptoms but also from their awareness that they might not survive it. Ramona Moll was hospitalized for COVID-19, which she believes she contracted on the front lines. She told NPR, "It's a very lonely feeling that you're going to die and you can't even say goodbye to your family." She also reported that she spent hours in isolation wondering: "I'm going to leave my daughter? I'm going to leave my husband? Who's going to take care of my daughter better than me?"[26]

Don Goepfert, an EMT in New York City, described feeling body aches after a shift and leaving the door open in case EMTs had to get in. He said, "I had that anxiety in me. . . . What if I don't make it through the next day? So I was trying to prepare for the worst." Later he, too, was admitted to the hospital.[27]

THEY ARE TERRIFIED OF BRINGING COVID-19 HOME TO THEIR LOVED ONES

After working in conditions that expose them to COVID-19 for hours at a time, healthcare workers are desperate not to bring the virus home to their family members. They go to great lengths to avoid their aging parents and do as much as they can to shield their spouses and children from the virus. Many families with a parent working in healthcare have packed up their children and sent them to live with relatives who are social distancing. Other healthcare workers have opted to sleep in different parts of the house, or even move out altogether.

Dr. Timmy Cheng, an Irvine pulmonary and critical care specialist, moved into a tent inside his family's garage to protect them from the coronavirus. He wrote on Facebook, "I voluntarily became homeless to protect my family should I become infected and bring the virus home."[28]

Those who must continue living at home go to extreme measures to stop the spread of the virus. They strip off their work clothes the moment they get home and drop them in the laundry. They spray their shoes and other personal items with disinfectant and shower obsessively. Despite this, they and their families live with the discomfort of knowing that exposure could happen at any moment.

THEY TAKE IT PERSONALLY WHEN COLLEAGUES GET SICK OR DIE (BECAUSE IT *IS* PERSONAL)

Healthcare providers have to detach somewhat to do their jobs. They witness trauma secondhand through their patients every day, but they can't fall apart because there is always another patient who needs help. But with COVID-19, not only do healthcare providers witness far more death and chaos than normal, but they are at risk of receiving the same fate. They have watched helplessly as their work colleagues get sick and sometimes even die. It is impossible to keep a stiff upper lip when the patient you are treating is your own teammate. That makes it personal. And it hurts.

Dr. Calvin Sun, an emergency and attending physician working throughout New York City, grieves the residents who have died. Those residents were "people in training that we were supposed to protect," he said. "That's like burying our own children."[29]

And unfortunately, some healthcare workers lost their lives to suicide during the pandemic. As previously mentioned, the entire medical community was shaken by the news of Dr. Lorna M. Breen's death.[30] Also in April 2020, John Mondello, an EMT with the FDNY, died by suicide. He had just started his career in January.[31] In a field already at risk for suicide, COVID-19 has shone a light on the need for greater mental health support for vulnerable healthcare workers.

THEY LOSE FAMILY MEMBERS TO COVID-19

Dr. Andrew Cohen is an emergency medicine physician at St. Joseph's University Medical Center. In March 2020 Dr. Cohen's mother-in-law, who lived in the same household, died from COVID-19. On the morning of her funeral, Dr. Cohen's father-in-law died as well. As he mourned, Dr. Cohen shared with the *New York Times* that he wonders,

"Did I bring this virus into my house?" He worries that he could be the next person in his household to succumb and performs an "over-the-top" cleansing ritual to help alleviate his fears and anxieties.[32]

THEY TREAT—AND LOSE—MEMBERS OF THEIR COMMUNITIES

Healthcare workers do not always treat people who are unknown to them. Sometimes their COVID-19 patients are beloved members of their own community. The *Wall Street Journal* reported this touching story:

Dr. Ivan Melendez, who works in Hidalgo County, Texas, received a video sent to him by his patient's son, telling his mother that he loves her. She was hospitalized with COVID-19. As he watched, another text came in from the son. "Mom died at 11:07. Were you able to show her my video?" Hours later,

> Dr. Melendez paused in the curtained room of the patient whose son had texted him that she died hours earlier. The deceased woman was his own mother's best friend, whom he had known since he was five. He slowly drew down the zipper of her body bag partway. He leaned down. He played the son's video saying a final "I love you." Then he gently zipped the bag up again and secured it with a rubber band.[33]

THEY ARE FRUSTRATED BECAUSE SOME PEOPLE *STILL* DO NOT TAKE COVID-19 SERIOUSLY

While healthcare providers fight to save patients from the deadly virus, they are shocked and upset by the many citizens not taking the pandemic seriously. Media coverage has shown packed beaches and parks, crowded holiday gatherings, and people attending crowded events as if nothing is wrong.

Some refuse to wear masks because they feel it infringes on their rights. Others insist that the virus is just an overhyped flu or even a political hoax or conspiracy. Whatever their reasons, this dismissive behavior is a slap in the face to those risking their own lives and the lives of their families to keep people safe.

Olumide Peter Kolade, a nurse from California who spent more than three months treating patients in New York, told the *New York Times*, "A few times I've lost my temper. . . . When someone tells me that they don't believe the virus is real, it's an insult. I take it personally."[34]

THEY FEEL HELPLESS SEEING COVID-19'S DEVASTATING TOLL ON VULNERABLE POPULATIONS

Healthcare providers are frustrated by the local governments' decisions to reopen communities too quickly and loosen the rules. This has a huge negative impact on low-income populations, who may have less access to information and might believe that it is safe to return to normal activities. Further, these groups are more likely to work in essential jobs, to house many generations in one home, and to have health conditions that put them at risk. Certain groups are overrepresented in COVID-19 infections. According to the Centers for Disease Control and Prevention (CDC), Non-Hispanic American Indian or Alaska Native persons have an age-adjusted hospitalization rate approximately five times that of non-Hispanic white persons; non-Hispanic black persons have a rate approximately five times that of non-Hispanic white persons; and Hispanic or Latino persons have a rate approximately four times that of non-Hispanic white persons.[35]

Doctors feared that the Rio Grande Valley along the US–Mexico border could see a massive surge of COVID-19 cases. "Much of the low-income population is employed in jobs that don't allow work from home, diabetes and obesity are common, and multigenerational households are the norm."[36]

THEY FEAR REPERCUSSIONS FOR SPEAKING OUT

Many employees in the healthcare industry have been hesitant to be critical of those in power for fear of losing their jobs. And some suffered consequences for speaking up. President Trump replaced Christi A. Grimm, the principal deputy inspector general at the Department of Health and Human Services, after her department released a survey finding that hospitals generally lacked supplies and equipment to prepare for the pandemic.[37] Dr. Nichole Quick is another example. She voluntarily resigned from her position as Orange County's chief health officer after defending her countywide face-mask order. The order was passionately opposed, and Dr. Quick even received what officials deemed to be a death threat.[38]

THEY ARE EXHAUSTED DUE TO PERSONNEL SHORTAGES

While most of the focus has been on equipment shortages, healthcare workers have been deeply impacted by staff shortages as increasing coronavirus cases boost demand. Having the specialized nurses, doctors, and other medical staff to deal with the way the virus manifests in patients is of utmost importance. But when hospitals lack these workers, everyone suffers. The existing staff are quickly overworked, patient care declines, and outcomes suffer. This only increases the overall strain felt by everyone.

As states experienced these shortages, government leaders called for help. On March 30, 2020, Michigan governor Gretchen Whitmer posted a video to Twitter, saying, "If you're a health professional anywhere in America, Michigan needs you. We're calling on doctors, and nurses, and respiratory therapists, and other health professionals to sign up and help us fight COVID-19 and save lives." New York governor Andrew Cuomo also put out a call for out-of-state doctors and nurses: "Help New York. We are the ones who are hit now."[39]

THEY ARE DEALING WITH THE BREAKDOWN AND SIDELINING OF LONG-RESPECTED GLOBAL AND GOVERNMENT ENTITIES

The institutions healthcare workers rely on have faced trials, missteps, and the loss of much of their power during the pandemic. This has left healthcare workers (and the rest of the country) unsure of what to believe or who to listen to and frustrated by their wavering positions and lack of power.

For example, when the first COVID-19 case appeared in the US, instead of using a ready-made test developed by the WHO, the CDC chose to create its own test, which malfunctioned and led to a series of delays.[40] Meanwhile, the CDC has wavered in its position on topics such as whether the public should wear masks or how to safely open restaurants and houses of worship.[41]

The WHO has also made errors. Instead of warning the world of the dangers of COVID-19 in a timely manner, the WHO stuck close to China's official positions, including its cover-ups.[42] (However, they may have been kept in the dark, as China gave the minimal amount of information required by law.[43])

Yet even despite these missteps, most healthcare professionals maintain a level of trust in these authorities. This is why so many have been upset when these authorities' influence is overridden. Specifically, in July 2020 the CDC was sidelined when hospitals were ordered to bypass the CDC and to send their COVID-19 data directly to the Department of Health and Human Services.[44] Also, after criticizing the WHO, President Trump announced that he would halt their funding.[45]

THEY FACE DECIMATED HOSPITAL BUDGETS FROM THE DROP IN ELECTIVE SURGERIES, AND MANY HAVE BEEN FURLOUGHED

Hospitals across the country are struggling with depleted revenue streams. Non-urgent surgeries were put on hold during lockdowns. The CDC reported that emergency department visits declined 42 percent during the early COVID-19 pandemic, from a mean of 2.1 million per week (March 31 to April 27, 2019) to 1.2 million (March 29 to April 25, 2020).[46]

And despite the shortage of doctors trained to deal with COVID-19 in various hotspots, a massive amount of healthcare employees are out of work. In April 2020, 1.4 million healthcare personnel lost their jobs, compared to 42,000 in March. Nearly 135,000 of the April losses were in hospitals.[47]

Fae-Marie Donathan, a per diem nurse in the Surgical ICU at the University of Cincinnati Medical Center, believed her skills would be essential. But as the pandemic took hold she was told she would no longer be scheduled. "I was thinking maybe I would have to worry about when I was going to get a day off," Donathan shared with NPR.

"I was thinking totally the opposite, never ever suspecting that I would be sitting at home not getting any hours at work."[48]

EXPERTS FEEL DEMORALIZED WHEN SCIENTIFIC FACT FALLS ON DEAF EARS

Infectious disease experts working in public health are stressed to the limit by the country and its leadership ignoring their warnings. Krutika Kuppalli, an infectious-disease physician, said, "I feel like I have been making the same recommendations since January." According to the *Atlantic*, experts feel "demoralized about repeatedly shouting evidence-based advice into a political void." Colin Carlson, a research professor at Georgetown University who specializes in infectious disease, said, "It feels like writing 'Bad things are about to happen' on a napkin and then setting the napkin on fire."[49]

After reading the many realities for healthcare workers in this chapter, it is clear that they have carried a heavy burden throughout this pandemic. Any one of these factors could be perceived as a traumatizing experience. When several are combined, they create a very real threat to a person's mental, emotional, and physical well-being.

The remainder of this book is dedicated to helping healthcare workers understand and process the fear and pain they are enduring. It is for anyone struggling with the aftermath of trauma or who has developed post-traumatic stress because of their experiences. If this describes you, take comfort. There is hope. Over the following chapters, we will talk about PTSD and how it develops, and we will lay out a roadmap for recovery.

CHAPTER 3

THE AFTERSHOCKS
ARE COMING

Stressful, traumatic experiences are nothing new for healthcare providers. It is a grueling industry that physically and emotionally grinds on its employees. Many in healthcare work long hours, experience sleep loss from being on call, and have limited free time to "fill the well." They also face more than their share of psychological demands, including the constant pressure to save lives, grief after losing patients, encounters with tragedy, and fighting against cynicism and futility in the presence of so much death.

These factors and others contribute to high instances of burnout and suicide. For example, the American College of Emergency Physicians shares that even before the pandemic, about 60 percent of emergency physicians experienced burnout in their career.[1] And about four hundred physicians die by suicide every year.[2]

Moral injury, mentioned in the last chapter, also contributes to their suffering. In the August 2018 issue of STAT News, Dr. Simon Talbot and Dr. Wendy Dean named moral injury as the true cause of burnout in healthcare—the cynicism, emotional or physical exhaustion, and diminished productivity that can be prevalent in many healthcare organizations.[3] And in the previous chapter, we saw first-hand the damage that moral injury has done to those on the front lines during COVID-19.

Burnout—and the factors leading to burnout—is a serious problem in healthcare, even in the best of times. Doctors, nurses, and all those working in the medical field are vulnerable to mental health issues like anxiety, depression, and substance abuse. But with COVID-19 in the picture, things go from bad to worse.

What is happening now with COVID-19 is bigger than burnout. Colin West, an internist who has studied physician well-being at the Mayo Clinic for more than fifteen years, said, "Burnout is a chronic response to health care conditions. This is an unprecedented acute crisis."[4]

To fight back against COVID-19, healthcare workers have had to work harder, faster, and longer than ever before (and this is already a group of people who pride themselves on working hard, long hours). They have seen a massive uptick in patient mortality and have been helpless to stop it. They've been terrified to go to work because the deadly virus is highly contagious, and PPE is in short supply. And they've been forced to make life-and-death triage decisions due to massive equipment shortages.

When you take a group of workers already dealing with high amounts of burnout and add the many forms of moral injury that make them feel like soldiers in a war, PTSD is a predictable outcome. If they have not already started experiencing post-traumatic stress, the wave is likely to hit once they have had time to reflect. That means the healthcare industry may have a serious mental health crisis on its hands in the near future. COVID-19 was the earthquake. Widespread cases of PTSD in healthcare providers are the aftershocks.

History has shown us that PTSD occurs in healthcare workers following epidemics.

HEALTHCARE WORKERS WERE TRAUMATIZED FOLLOWING THE SARS 2003 OUTBREAK AND EBOLA 2014-16 OUTBREAK

Let's examine how the SARS outbreak in 2003 and the Ebola outbreaks that started in 2014 have impacted healthcare workers.

- During the SARS epidemic of 2003, 89 percent of the 271 healthcare workers in Hong Kong reported negative psychological effects, including exhaustion and fear of social contact.[5]
- Out of 549 randomly selected employees of a hospital in Beijing, 10 percent of the respondents had experienced high levels of post-traumatic stress symptoms since the SARS outbreak. Respondents who had been quarantined, or who worked in high-risk locations such as SARS wards—or those who had friends or close relatives who had contracted SARS—were two to three times more likely to have high post-traumatic stress symptom levels.[6]
- And for up to two years following the epidemic, healthcare workers in Toronto, another city hit hard by SARS, had significantly higher levels of burnout, psychological distress, and post-traumatic stress.[7]
- The more recent Ebola outbreaks in 2014–16 also mirror the trauma that healthcare workers are experiencing with COVID-19, including watching their colleagues get sick and die, persevering in terrifying circumstances, worrying about their own well-being, and being isolated from their support systems.[8]

PTSD SYMPTOMS MAY ALREADY BE OCCURRING IN HEALTHCARE WORKERS

Early research indicates that healthcare workers are experiencing PTSD symptoms. In May 2020 JAMA Network Open published a survey of 1,257 healthcare workers in thirty-four hospitals across China. It was found that by early February, 72 percent had experienced symptoms of distress. About half had symptoms of depression and anxiety. Over one-third had insomnia. Shaohua Hu, a psychiatrist at the First Affiliated Hospital of the Zhejiang University School of Medicine who conducted the study, reported that the main reason for distress at the beginning of the outbreak was the lack of PPE.[9]

The writing is on the wall. If you are a healthcare provider on the front lines of this pandemic, unfortunately you may be at risk of developing post-traumatic stress. While no one can stop the pandemic or protect you from the frightening and distressing experiences you encounter on the job, what we *can* give you is hope. Because there are many tools out there to help you process everything you have been through and start to heal.

In the next chapter we will take a closer look at trauma and lay out the 12 Phases Emotional Algorithm and identify other mental health issues that occur alongside PTSD. And in later chapters we will explore some of the things you can do to find relief.

CHAPTER 4

THE PATH TO PTSD

DR. MARK GOULSTON

First, let's define PTSD, or Post-Traumatic Stress Disorder. PTSD is a serious disorder that occurs in people who have witnessed or survived traumatic, terrifying, shocking, or dangerous experiences. On the surface people with PTSD might appear to be healthy, happy, and functioning. But in reality they are struggling to survive and are nowhere near being able to thrive.

People with PTSD face disabling symptoms, including a hyper-alert nervous system, detachment, numbness, flashbacks, and intrusive thoughts, and sometimes they struggle with depression or substance abuse. Naturally, this can impact their ability to establish or sustain meaningful relationships, continue going to work each day, and reach their goals.

Thankfully, you do not have to suffer and live with debilitating symptoms for the rest of your life. PTSD is treatable. Most people are able to reduce their symptoms, reclaim the peace and happiness they lost, and resume their whole and healthy lives.

WHAT IS TRAUMA?

Before we can look at how PTSD manifests step by step, we need to better understand trauma, because trauma is what causes PTSD. And to be clear, trauma is different from stress. Everyone—particularly those in healthcare—deals with stress every day, and most people are able to manage routine stress in the moment and move on.

Trauma, however, is defined as a deeply distressing, disturbing, and overwhelming event that threatens your life or the lives of people around you. It is often something unexpected that catches you by surprise, is horrifying and terrifying, and causes you to feel fear, helplessness, and lack of control. Experiencing trauma often shatters your previous sense of safety and security. It can change the way you look at the world. And it can create lasting harm.

Based on this description it is understandable why, as a healthcare worker, you may be struggling to handle your work life during the pandemic. The trauma of COVID-19 is vast and multilayered. And unlike regular citizens who primarily fear for their own lives and their loved ones, as frontline workers you bear the burden of putting yourself in harm's way while seeing firsthand the terrifying impact of the virus each time you go to work.

THE 12 PHASES EMOTIONAL ALGORITHM: THE ROAD TO, THROUGH, AND BACK FROM TRAUMA

You may be wondering how PTSD develops in the first place. Below is a framework I developed to describe the processes that typically occur in your psyche when a traumatic experience takes place. While the twelve phases take into account the experiences of healthcare providers facing the COVID-19 pandemic, they also apply to anyone experiencing trauma so intensely that it may lead to PTSD. Phases one through ten describe everything that occurs from the time the trauma occurs to the time when PTSD develops. Phases eleven and twelve—which I touch on here and will delve into more in chapter 5—highlight the journey to recovery and, finally, healing.

1. **TRAUMA**—This is an event of vast proportions that shocks, distresses, and overwhelms you beyond any stressful experience you have ever had, or ever imagined you could handle, which temporarily causes you to fight, flee, or freeze mentally and physically.

2. **HORROR**—You see or experience horrific things without having the opportunity to fully feel the horror. This also includes unexpected shock, surprise, and the inability to comprehend what's happening or catch up to your visual/auditory senses. This typically applies to traumas consisting of a single event, but it also applies to the horror of seeing much more death than expected, witnessing people gasping for breath and dying alone, and other horrifying events occurring during the pandemic. Accompanying this and triggered by your pituitary gland is a huge outpouring of cortisol from your adrenal glands that signals, "Get—physically—ready, you're in danger."

3. **TERROR**—You feel that your mere existence is becoming increasingly precarious and your primary focus becomes the survival of your body and psyche. During this phase you experience an involuntary biological reaction that includes the fight/flight/freeze responses that occur when a person is in danger. Your highly elevated cortisol signals the amygdala part of your brain (your "emotional sentinel") to divert blood flow away from your upper, rational thinking brain to your lower, survival brain. This has been referred to as an Amygdala Hijack.

By the way, something that mitigates the intensity is having colleagues also going through this—esprit de corps—which causes an increase in oxytocin and bonding that makes the terror more tolerable and manageable through the trauma. In wartime, soldiers will often say they didn't panic and run, even though they wanted to, because they couldn't let their fellow soldiers down who felt similarly toward them. That can be the temporizing effect of powerfully and collectively felt oxytocin, the hormone associated with emotional connectedness and emotional safety. Oxytocin counteracts high cortisol and can partially stave off a full Amygdala Hijack, but the continued stress can overtake this.

4. **FRAGILE**—In spite of the benefit of going through this trauma with a "fire team"—your colleagues fighting by your side in the battle against COVID-19—when you're on your own, you may feel like a windshield in a car that has become cracked, yet not broken. You are likely to feel that the next hit to the windshield will cause it to shatter and that you will never come back. What has shattered is your prior belief system about safety and security, which allowed you to go through your everyday life.

What once seemed outside the boundaries of reasonable or expected but still manageable, no longer is. It's like a bubble of protection has popped. Groundlessness and uncertainty dominate—and the struggle thereafter to reestablish the bubble or eventually construct a new framework, one that encompasses the new reality of potential risk, seems impossible. This can trigger a state of free-floating anxiety that verges on panic at any moment. And if panic sets in, you think you have lost your mind and that it will never return.

5. **OVERRIDING PANIC**—Being duty bound by your work causes you to clamp down on any feelings to avoid becoming overwhelmed and freezing as you see others in need and hurting,

and as you feel your own helplessness and powerlessness. You may want to lash out and blame others as well.

6. **SUPPRESSED THOUGHTS**—You consciously push whatever you're tempted to think about out of your conscious mind in order to focus, which rapidly becomes exhausting. Life goes on, but the horror and terror compounded by the guilt, shame, or blame you feel don't get fully processed. Why? Because these are too psychologically dangerous to broach. Over time this tendency to suppress your thoughts may increase because you believe that your thoughts will only make a bad situation worse or that they are a personal weakness.

7. **REPRESSED FEELINGS**—You don't have as much conscious control over your feelings as you do over your thoughts. Fortunately, and for the sake of survival, your mind pushes the feelings further down into your unconscious and away from your conscious mind, so it does not take as much energy to keep them away. However, this may produce compulsive behaviors such as overeating, drinking, exhaustion, irritability, or withdrawal outside of work.

Concomitantly, positive coping measures focused on growth that (seemingly) keep the feelings at bay are palliative at best. Though healthy, these actions don't relieve or resolve the root issue. For example, one positive coping mechanism that may help in the short term but not in the long term is to focus on becoming even more skilled in something to make you feel more in control in your job. Something else that further enables you to repress your feelings is the adrenaline rush you feel from the fear and even the excitement from all the danger you're facing. Adrenaline, however, is like "fool's bold," causing you to superficially believe you're doing fine when down deep you know you're not. All of this occurs at the expense of self-care—like spending even more time reading and learning until 2:00 a.m. when you're already sleep deprived, when you would do better to improve your sleep and/or practice meditation or yoga.

8. **FOCUS AND FUNCTION**—You focus and carry on. This is what you now do to live up to responsibilities because there is a higher need at the moment to lead, organize, and unify. There is no time to process meaning-making unless it is limited to unifying, mission-critical, and mission-centric activities. You must attend to first things first and will deal with feelings later.

9. **DANGER HAS PASSED**—When an acute threat has passed, instead of being able to fully relax, you may internally relax your guard that has protected you from experiencing intolerable feelings. However, with that internal guard lowered, horror and terror now threaten to push up through the cumulative vulnerability that built up inside you. It caused you to feel that something inside wasn't right even as you were functioning and running on adrenaline to your and other's amazement. However, the unfelt feelings you repressed and pushed away while the trauma was occurring can now come out and may even cause you to feel as if you might explode or shatter. Sadly and tragically for some, this is when thoughts of suicide surface as a preferred option, rather than believe you could lose total control (which is a part of your identity), fall apart, and never come back.

Imagine the analogy of an abscess that is not fully drained and instead sutured prematurely. At any time, a small infection could worsen. When that happens, that abscess can grow into a fulminating wound that threatens to burst and cause sepsis. This leads to retriggering/activation, especially for you who remain in the same setting where the trauma occurred and feel as if your repressed thoughts and feelings could also break through inside you and cause psychological sepsis, a.k.a. the feeling that you are losing your mind. Your logical, rational mind may say, *I'm safe*, but your body says, *You're lying*. This is especially true if and when additional threats emerge in the same setting. Keep in mind that as a healthcare worker, you will likely continue to return to the scene of the trauma each time you go to work, so it is very normal to experience hypervigilance—a state of increased alertness. Until you are able to process everything you have gone through, the body will continue to override the mind.

10. **PTSD**—As we reviewed earlier, post-traumatic stress disorder causes many disabling and upsetting symptoms. When repressed feelings push to come out, they threaten to eviscerate your psyche because you don't know how you survived the trauma in the first place, and you don't believe you can survive it a second time. In fact, if you say to such people, "Good for you, you're so strong, you got over that," they will not infrequently tell you, "I never got over it. I got past it. And I don't know how I did and I don't think I could make it through it again."

11. **DISABLED OR RECOVERED**—We will explore this step more in the next chapter, but this is the point at which a person either becomes further impaired by the trauma they experienced or embarks on a journey to healing.

12. **HEALED**—Finally the person fully reexperiences the trauma, along with the full spectrum of emotions and feelings the trauma created, and regains the capacity to feel peace and joy at last. It is as if in finishing thinking what you wouldn't allow yourself to think and finishing feeling what you left unfelt, the abscess fully drains and heals from the inside out—and you are guided through that process with empathy from others. This empathy enables you to remain calm enough to listen to and follow solutions that lasted. We will focus on the healing process in chapters 5 and 6.

———

While you may feel overwhelmed or upset reading over this 12 Phases Emotional Algorithm, do not despair. In chapter 5 you will learn how to empathically revisit each step you see above, attach the unfelt emotions and feelings, and process the traumatic events that are causing you pain. But for now, we will focus on the experience of having PTSD.

THREE LEVELS OF REACTIONS TO TRAUMA

When a traumatic event or a traumatic series of events takes place, a person will respond to the stress induced by trauma in one of three ways:

- a short-term reaction to the stress,
- a period of acute stress, or
- PTSD.

After a *stress response* to typical stressors/mild traumas, you may have anxiety, fear, shock, grief, or a feeling of numbness that lasts for days, weeks, or months. You may notice an increased startle response, trouble sleeping, or headache. You could also have difficulty concentrating or remembering the stressful event. These stress reactions typically fade as time passes.

But sometimes the symptoms, feelings, or emotions last longer—and due to the unprecedented, extraordinary circumstances surrounding COVID-19, we expect many more people to struggle even when they haven't struggled with past traumas. If this happens you may be experiencing *acute stress disorder*, characterized by more severe symptoms, including dissociation (feeling dazed, spaced out, numb, or as if the world is unreal). Acute stress disorder can also cause anxiety and hypervigilance, along with a desire to avoid anything associated with the trauma. If you experience the symptoms of acute stress disorder for a month or longer, your condition may then meet the diagnostic criteria for PTSD.

SYMPTOMS OF PTSD

PTSD shows up in several ways, including:

- intrusive thoughts,
- avoidance,
- negative thoughts, and
- hyperarousal.

Intrusive Thoughts

People with PTSD continue to reexperience the trauma through unwanted and upsetting memories, nightmares, flashbacks, emotional distress, and physical reactivity after exposure to reminders of the trauma. Intrusive thoughts are unwelcome thoughts or memories that appear over and over and commonly appear as flashbacks to the traumatizing event. While we all have unpleasant thoughts from time to time, these are particularly difficult to brush aside. They can cause extremely uncomfortable emotions, such as fear, anger, helplessness, and humiliation.

Avoidance

People with PTSD also develop avoidance habits to protect themselves from the pain and to make their distressing thoughts and feelings go away. They may avoid returning to the place the trauma occurred or avoid anything that reminds them of the trauma. (Which, in this case, is a problem!)

Negative Thoughts

In addition to these powerful and haunting memories and sensations, people may also develop negative thoughts that stem from the trauma, such as "I'm not a good doctor/nurse/paramedic" or "I didn't do enough to save my patient" or "I'm not a good mother/father because I am exposing my children to the virus." They may be unable to recall key features of the trauma, become disinterested in social activities and isolated from others, and have difficulty experiencing joy and happiness.

Hyperarousal

Finally, people with PTSD show signs of hyperarousal, during which their nervous systems stay on alert to help them stay safe. As previously said, since they believe that they won't survive another similar trauma, hyperarousal keeps them constantly on the lookout for anything that might reactivate their trauma and become that second shoe they are afraid will drop. This can lead to irritability, anger, edginess, and exhaustion. They may have heart palpitations, sweaty palms, and difficulty resting or relaxing.

Hyperarousal can also cause panic attacks. Panic attacks occur when you have sudden, intense fear. They are not dangerous, but you may feel as if you are dying or losing control during a panic attack. Some symptoms include sweating, a fast heartbeat, difficulty breathing, shallow breathing, feeling faint, and the urge to scream or run away.

To read more about the diagnostic criteria from the *Diagnostic and Statistical Manual of Mental Disorders* (DSM-5), visit this site: https://www.ptsd.va.gov/professional/treat/essentials/dsm5_ptsd.asp.

If you believe you may be experiencing symptoms of post-traumatic stress, visit the following site for a screening tool: https://www.ptsd.va.gov/professional/assessment/screens/pc-ptsd.asp. While this assessment can give you valuable insight, do not attempt to self-diagnose

PTSD. Instead, seek diagnosis from a medical professional such as a psychologist, a psychiatrist, or your primary care doctor. They can take your medical and personal history into account along with other criteria before making a diagnosis.

A WORD ON COMPLEX PTSD

There are two types of PTSD, simple and complex. Simple PTSD generally occurs after a single event such as a natural disaster or an accident. Complex PTSD occurs when a person with an already traumatized core (often stemming from ongoing childhood abuse of some sort, but sometimes stemming from trauma related to war, chronic domestic abuse, etc.) faces new trauma in adulthood. When this happens, it not only traumatizes the person from the outside in, it also reactivates their old unhealed trauma from the inside out. In essence, they got *past* the trauma, but they never got *over* it.

If you have complex PTSD, your healing process might look slightly different from a person with simple PTSD. Working with a therapist can often help if it seems your feelings of vulnerability surpass that which can be fully explained by the recent trauma.

OTHER PSYCHIATRIC PROBLEMS THAT SOMETIMES OCCUR ALONGSIDE PTSD

PTSD can cause new mental health issues in patients who didn't have those issues prior to their trauma or it can worsen the symptoms of preexisting mental disorders. A few of these psychological disorders include depression, anxiety disorders, alcohol or drug abuse, eating disorders, and self-injury.

Depression

Up to half of those with PTSD show enough symptoms to also be diagnosed with depression or major depressive disorder. In addition to the changes that PTSD has on the brain's biochemistry and structure, PTSD creates roadblocks for careers, relationships, and life in general. And sad life events increase the risk for depression. Symptoms of depression include: hopelessness, insomnia or oversleeping, sadness, apathy, trouble thinking or concentrating, suicidal thoughts or actions, feelings of worthlessness, loss of interest in everyday activities, and anxiety and agitation.

Anxiety Disorders

When symptoms of anxiety are severe enough or fall into a specific category, you may be diagnosed with an anxiety disorder. Some of them include:

- *Generalized Anxiety.* Having persistent, excessive worry about a range of topics.
- *Agoraphobia.* The fear or inability to leave your home or go more than a short distance from your home. People with agoraphobia have trouble feeling safe in public places.
- *Panic Disorder.* Having sudden and repeated disabling attacks of fear lasting for several minutes or longer (panic attacks).
- *Obsessive-Compulsive Disorder (OCD).* People with OCD have uncontrollable recurring thoughts (obsessions) and/or behaviors (compulsions) that they feel the urge to repeat over and over. Examples include constantly checking to see if the front door is locked or worrying obsessively over germs.
- *Social Phobia,* also known as *Social Anxiety Disorder.* This is defined as an extreme fear of being around other people in everyday situations. People with this phobia fear being watched and judged by others.

Alcohol and/or Drug Abuse

People with PTSD show high rates of alcohol dependence and drug abuse due to the pain, anxiety, and suffering associated with the disorder. PTSD sufferers turn to alcohol or drugs to numb the overwhelming feelings they experience regularly. While these substances can temporarily soothe the pain of trauma, keep nightmares at bay, and ease the discomfort of social situations, it is not a healthy way to cope.

Eating Disorders

People suffering from PTSD sometimes use food to cope with painful feelings and emotions associated with their trauma. Eating disorders give them a sense of control, a distraction from problems a person does not want to face, and immediate, though temporary, relief.

A person with PTSD may show signs of *bulimia nervosa*. In this disorder a person binges on food, then vomits, or exercises excessively, or takes laxatives to avoid gaining weight. Some people with PTSD also compulsively overeat, a disorder known as *binge eating disorder*. It's no coincidence that a number of foods, especially the unhealthy yet tasty ones that people overindulge in, are referred to as "comfort foods."

Another eating disorder, *anorexia nervosa*, occurs when a person stops eating sufficiently for their energy needs for fear of weight gain.

Self-Injury

Sometimes people with PTSD engage in self-harming behaviors. These behaviors can include cutting, burning, needle-sticking, head-banging, biting, scratching, or punching oneself. People who engage in self-injury do so for many reasons. It makes them feel something (especially if they are numb); it creates a sense of control; it creates an endorphin-fueled emotional high (endorphins are feel-good chemicals that dampen emotional pain); it is a way for them to punish themselves; it is a cry for help; it is a way to dissociate.

Now you not only know what PTSD looks like, you also know some of the other mental health issues that hitch a ride alongside PTSD. You may be surprised to recognize some of your own behaviors described above. If so, you don't have to suffer through debilitating symptoms or figure things out on your own.

Our advice for anyone struggling with these symptoms is to seek help and work with a therapist to get the right diagnosis (or diagnoses) to begin shining a light on the feelings and emotions that are causing you pain.

Of course, many in healthcare may hesitate to get help when they need it most. Why? Because of the longstanding stigma against mental illnesses such as PTSD in our society.

THE STIGMA OF PTSD

It is well known that there is a stigma around PTSD. To the outside world, you might *appear* to be okay. So when you struggle, people might not understand why. They may even believe things are all in your head, or that you should just be able to move on. This is not surprising given our country's just-get-over-it culture, which we discussed in chapter 1. This same culture has impacted the healthcare industry as employees pride themselves on being able to perform under stressful, tiring, and often upsetting circumstances. When a healthcare worker can't just get over it, they may not receive much patience from others.

Further, those who do understand the potential severity of PTSD may keep you at arm's length. They might label you with stereotypes such as *unpredictable* or *moody*. This only contributes to the problem. And sadly, the person suffering often feels their own internalized shame for struggling as well.

Let us remind you that fight-flight-freeze is a normal biological reaction to trauma. And for many, the trauma of COVID-19 is overwhelming in so many ways and it is not surprising to feel the way you do. So do not take on extra suffering because of the stigma of PTSD.

The emerging nomenclature around PTSD expresses the idea that it should be thought of not so much as a mental *disorder* (and therefore something pathological) but rather as a mental *injury*. This is an important mental shift, especially for those who might resist an unwanted diagnosis and not seek the help they need.

Throughout this book we have used the term PTSD because this is the name the public is most familiar with. However, we look forward to the day when patients and healthcare providers alike will embrace the alternate title: Post Traumatic Stress Injury or PTSI. This will further remove the stigma people feel around this serious health injury and empower people to get help when they need it.

In chapter 5 we will cover the therapeutic treatment options that can bring relief.

CHAPTER 5

THE ROAD BACK
FROM TRAUMA

DR. MARK GOULSTON

In the previous chapter we discussed the phases that lead to PTSD following a trauma. In this chapter we will learn about the pathway to recovery and available treatment options. But first let's take another look at the way PTSD develops.

To review, here is the 12 Phases Emotional Algorithm that leads to PTSD. As you can see below, once you have PTSD, you either recover or become further disabled.

1. Trauma
2. Horror
3. Terror
4. Fragile
5. Overriding Panic
6. Suppressed Thoughts
7. Repressed Feelings

8. Focus and Function
9. Danger Has Passed
10. PTSD
11. Disabled or Recovered
12. Healed

It's time to address the final two phases of this cycle: *Disabled or Recovered* and *Healed*. Here's what they mean.

DISABLED OR RECOVERED

Disabled

If you grow to be more disabled due to the traumas you have endured, things can rapidly go from bad to worse. Assuming that a fire team is not established so that a person can safely debrief their experiences and find understanding, that person may instead isolate and try to numb themselves in various ways (for example, with alcohol or drugs).

Meanwhile their trauma or traumas fester like an undrained abscess, and the unfelt and unprocessed emotions from the trauma push themselves through as nightmares or flashbacks. Individuals may develop hypervigilance in order to avoid any triggers that will threaten to reignite the horror/terror/panic trifecta that leads to psychological paralysis.

Keep in mind that this describes the worst-case scenario. Our goal is to circumvent this from happening, through therapy, group work, and exercises that help you process your experiences and heal. The flip side to being *disabled* is *recovered*. Read on to learn more.

Recovered

True recovery—breaking free from the parts of the trauma that hold you back—requires processing and accepting the trauma you have experienced and living with it as something that is not a bad dream but something that actually happened, but that is no longer happening in your life even if it seems to continue to happen in your mind. Just because you're afraid doesn't mean you're in any danger, but your mind may not believe what your body is still reacting to. The recovery process takes time and effort.

Of course, in the case of COVID-19 the threat is ongoing, and as a healthcare worker, you may in fact be in danger. Nonetheless, you can continually work toward processing traumatic experiences and memories so you can move out of survival mode and regain as much peace as possible.

In our society we confuse positive behaviors as evidence of recovery. But it's not enough to focus on positivity, gratitude, and the like and to believe that this positive focus means you are healed from PTSD. (That is simply putting "lipstick on a pain" and fails to address the wound of trauma itself.) Nor is it enough to treat the negative coping methods that many with PTSD develop, such as substance abuse or eating disorders, or even negative coping mechanisms that are perceived as positives in our society, such as workaholism. Recovery programs to treat these offshoots of PTSD are certainly important, but simply resolving those behaviors does not guarantee healing either.

The bottom line: true recovery is unlikely to happen without safely feeling the horror, terror, and fragile feelings you short-circuited and bypassed to survive and also addressing the blame, shame, and guilt that may be at the heart of the traumatic response.

HEALED

The final step is healing. Healing is defined as eliminating and, if possible, eradicating the intrusive symptoms of PTSD, including hypervigilance, nightmares, numbing, and compulsive self-defeating behaviors. To heal, your psyche must reexperience the trauma so that many of the emotions attached to the trauma are fully experienced and the unfelt feelings that you were not able to face are finally felt.

Remember the earlier image of suturing an abscess prematurely. Healing can't happen until the abscess is fully drained, allowing the natural healing that occurs from the inside out. It has been achieved when a state of mind and psyche exists where intrusive symptoms—including hypervigilance, nightmares, and psychological numbing—are either gone or rarely present. Instead of looking tentatively where you are going with excessive caution, you go where you are looking with a sense of curiosity and desire for adventure. Exhaustion is replaced by the capacity to feel peace and joy.

By now you understand that PTSD is a serious issue that you must address in order to heal. In the following pages we will delve into the treatments and exercises that can help you reclaim your life. You'll notice that the majority of these treatments revolve around therapy. Working with a therapist is an important component of healing. Later on we will cover tips on finding the right therapist, but for now we will explore some of the best treatment options out there.

TREATMENT OPTIONS

Surgical Empathy

Before covering the basics of some of the established treatment routes for PTSD, I would like to cover the approach I developed to help people heal from post-traumatic stress. I call it *surgical empathy*.

Surgical empathy is a wonderful healing modality to try when usual treatments are not fully reaching people. Sometimes a patient's mind is so overwhelmed from external stimuli and their internal suppressed, repressed, unfelt, unprocessed, and undealt-with pain, that a "surgical" approach is needed to meet them where they are and help them "feel felt" and less alone in their feelings.

To "feel felt" means to feel enveloped in the safety of being connected with someone in a way that almost immediately reduces hurt, fear, anxiety, and emotional pain. The relief that feeling of safety provides is often so powerful that many people spontaneously begin to cry.

Surgical empathy can break through to people stuck in irrational, nonfunctioning self-preservation through enabling them to talk out their doubts, fears, and blockages, empathizing with them rather than trying to convince them to see things another way. When people are stressed, their cortisol level is elevated. As you likely know, cortisol is secreted by the adrenal glands to help the body deal with stress after your pituitary gland has signaled it to do so. When your cortisol level goes up, it can lead to the amygdala becoming overactivated, causing an increase in blood flow to the lower fight-flight-freeze reptilian brain and away from our upper rational, listening, thinking brain— the aforementioned Amygdala Hijack. You are probably familiar with fight-or-flight—your body's natural stress response to threat in which you either fight to defend yourself or flee to safety. The freeze response is less widely known. When people are threatened by danger, and when fight or flight is not possible, people freeze as a means of survival. Freezing is much like playing dead in the animal kingdom. Much like animals in the wild, freezing makes us less of a target.

When a stressed person is empathized with and feels not just understood but felt, this leads to a release and sometimes a surge of oxytocin, which often induces crying from relief. This promotes bonding and closeness. When oxytocin goes up, cortisol goes down, the amygdala settles down, blood flow returns to the upper brain, and that previously stressed-out person can calm down and engage in a rational and constructive conversation.

Surgical empathy addresses the "abscess," or trauma, that many people live with, especially those suffering from PTSD. Imagine that you have a red and inflamed wound or abscess (a graphic image, yes, but a fitting one). There's no denying that the abscess is there, but if you try very hard you can almost forget about it. But when you happen to bump it . . . watch out! The pain is excruciating. Trapped trauma is a lot like that angry and painful abscess. However, through a surgically empathetic approach, it is possible to drain the abscess and alleviate the pain.

Surgical empathy works by tapping safely into what the patient is experiencing. When you are able to accurately pinpoint what a patient feels and they then confirm or express it to you, that patient feels less alone, less ashamed, less afraid, and calm enough to listen to reasonable solutions. To sum it up in a sentence: having horror heard helps heal hurt. (You can think of it at the Six *H*s.) When patients share their stories and feel felt, they can begin to heal.

What Makes Surgical Empathy Different

Until a person suffering from PTSD taps into their pain and feels felt, they may cope, but they will frequently not heal. If anyone were to push solutions or well-meaning advice on PTSD patients before their feelings have been fully felt, it is the equivalent to suturing an abscess too soon. Instead of healing, the wound risks becoming septic.

There is a dramatic analogy to how quick solutions may work temporarily to distract from symptoms, but they only lead to PTSD later. In the COVID-19 pandemic many states in America opened too soon and provided immediate relief to the isolation and business standstill caused by pervasive "stay at home/shelter in place" orders, but reopening led to widespread surges of cases and deaths. In the case of COVID-19, the wound had not had time to heal completely, and premature attempts to reopen communities unleashed more trauma on the country.

This is a subtle but significant difference between clinical empathy and surgical empathy.

Clinical empathy—*I can understand how and why you might be feeling a, b, and c.* This type of approach validates but keeps an intellectual and clinical distance from the patient.

Surgical empathy—*I sense that you're feeling a, b, and c. Is that true?* (They answer.)
At its worst, how awful does that get for you? (They answer.)
Will you tell me about one of those "at its worst" times? (They answer.)
When that happened, how did you feel? (They answer.)
What did it make you want to do to try to feel better? (They answer.)
How did that work out? (They answer.)
If, going forward, you get into another one of those states, what would be a better thing to do? (They answer.)
Why is that? (They answer.)
Would you do me a favor? The next time you get into such a place, can you either text me or a friend or family member and tell them, or try what you just said and then text me how that worked out? (They answer.)

To practice surgical empathy, you have to set your personal agenda aside and go deep into the hurt, fear, and despair (what I call *des-pair*, which I'll explain below) of another person in a way that causes them to finally feel felt. If you can let go of your "here" and wholeheartedly meet another person at their "there," you can open their mind to you. Because you've gone to their "there," you've narrowed the emotional gap between you and them, enabling them to lean toward and meet you there. This increases their oxytocin (closeness and relief from feeling alone) so they want more from you, which increases their dopamine (pleasure to counterbalance some of their pain).

A Deep Look at Des-pair

Let's take a moment to talk about the des-pair that a person may face after experiencing trauma. When a person is locked in the grips of PTSD, they can be driven to feeling des-pair, meaning they may feel *unpaired* with reasons to get themselves unstuck.

They feel:

- Unpaired with a future = hopeless
- Unpaired with an ability to help themselves = helpless
- Unpaired with any power to help themselves = powerless
- Unpaired with worth (if they can't accomplish anything) = worthless
- Unpaired with productivity or confidence that they contribute = useless
- Unpaired with meaning for life = meaningless
- Unpaired with any sense of purpose = purposeless
- Unpaired with the cumulative effects of all of the above = pointless

Because of their inability to pair with hope, help, worth, etc., some individuals suffering from PTSD will instead pair with death (by suicide), opiates, alcohol, or other vehicles of destruction in an attempt to make the pain go away.

Finding Your Fire Team: How Group Work Can Help You Recover from PTSD

Group work can be an effective tool during your healing journey. As a healthcare worker you are part of a team, whether you are a paramedic with the fire department, a nurse within a medical group, a

CNA within a nursing home system, an emergency room doctor at a hospital, or any other healthcare worker. While you experienced the countless traumas of the pandemic, the teammates by your side were going through the same experiences. People were traumatized en masse, and the steps to recovery can be accelerated if they are implemented en masse.

Why en masse?

Because just as fire teams in the military (and among first responders and healthcare providers) experience a trauma and work together to do what is necessary to survive that trauma, fire teams also need to be instituted so you can go through the full recovery from that trauma. Otherwise individuals often isolate and try to numb themselves. This frequently leads to PTSD.

This is why *your* fire team—fellow trauma survivors who lived through the same horror you experienced—can be such a powerful part of your healing. When groups share similar suppressed and repressed thoughts and feelings during and following a trauma, they are immersed in the bonding hormone, oxytocin.

Again, oxytocin is associated with emotional connectedness and emotional safety. It also counteracts high cortisol, the hormone released to deal with stress. Remember that when our minds and brains are under the effect of high cortisol, the emotional part of our brain called the amygdala signals blood flow to go preferentially to our lower, more primitive survival brain and away from our prefrontal, thinking, cortex (the Amygdala Hijack). However, when people experience a surge of oxytocin, cortisol decreases, their amygdalae settle down, blood flow returns to the prefrontal cortex, and they can again think rationally and think through their options.

Check if your organization already has a formal support group. If not, consider forming your own peer support group. You can meet once or twice a week for sessions in person or even by video conference call to share your fears, anxieties, struggles, and yes, even your victories. What's important is that you have a network of support when you need it most.

Below are surgical empathy exercises. Many can be done alone or in groups, and I have given instructions for individual exercises as well as for the group approach. No matter how you choose to apply them, these exercises can help you face your feelings and begin to process them.

As you move forward, be aware that participating in treatments or exercises that allow you to go through all the phases you skipped to survive your trauma might awaken feelings that seem to go beyond your present or recent traumatic situation. If this occurs, it is possible that your present feeling of vulnerability is stirring up something unresolved from your past. Rest assured that these feelings can be addressed, talked through, fully felt, and then released with a qualified therapist. Or, if you are going through the recovering and healing process as part of a fire team, it might be helpful for one of the members to ask the group, "Do any of you feel that the present/recent trauma is triggering prior traumas that a subgroup of us might want to share and talk through outside of the larger group?"

EXERCISE 1: DISTRESS RELIEF
EXERCISE AND JOURNAL

This distress relief exercise is a wonderful tool that you can use over and over to recognize your feelings and your reactions to your feelings anytime an upset (no matter how large or small) occurs. This tool is particularly useful when you feel triggered by anything that reminds you of the traumas of COVID-19, be it the noise of sirens, a COVID-related news story, the memory of a patient who died, etc.

When a trigger occurs, mentally walk yourself through the steps listed below.

- Date/Time: _____ / _____
- What just happened?
- What did you *think* when it happened?
- What did you *feel* when it happened?
- What does it *make* you want to do now?
- Take a deep breath.
- What would be a *better* thing to do now?
- Why is that better?

Take your time and mentally answer each question. First, recall what just happened that upset you so badly. Next, focus on what you thought and felt about the incident. Then think about what the incident made you want to do (sometimes distressing incidents make us want to do destructive things like fly into a rage, drink too many alcoholic drinks, or engage in self-harm). Before you do any of those things, pause and take a slow, deep breath. Next, think about something you could do instead that would be healthy and useful. Maybe you could stop what you are doing and take a ten-minute walk. Or continue breathing slowly and deeply for five minutes. Finally, answer the question, "Why is that better?" Why is the new solution a better or healthier solution?

If you are part of a support group, you can take turns recalling a triggering incident or upset that occurred recently and talking through the steps that led you (or could lead you next time) to a better outcome. Otherwise, you can continue to do this process alone each time.

Another great way to use this exercise is to create a journal. Each time you are in distress, write down your answers and insights to the questions. You can even include on the first page a photograph of a mentor, hero, coach, parent, or supportive friend, living or deceased. Imagine that they are the ones asking you these questions and supporting you as you continue to grow and heal. As you hear them talking and walking you through it, you will feel their love and belief in you.

This will cause a surge of oxytocin, which will counteract your high cortisol, and that will be followed by a release of dopamine as you feel your gratitude and appreciation toward that person.

EXERCISE 2: THE 12 WORDS

This is a powerful surgical empathy tool I use to help patients tap into their feelings when they are stuck or frozen due to trauma. Together we gently visit key words one at a time, which gives the patient time to identify with each emotion. As the patient does this within the safety of the conversation, it stops the Amygdala Hijack, and their mind is able to relax. From that relaxed state, they are able to think about rational next steps and solutions to further their healing.

You can do the 12 words exercise on your own, in therapy with your practitioner, or as part of a group exercise. If doing it on your own, imagine a trusted friend or loved one gently and empathetically guiding you through the exercise. If you are in a group, the moderator can lead the exercise by speaking each word to the group, or to a single individual in the group. You don't have to cover all the words at once. You can focus on just one or two words, take a break, and start on a new word later.

STEP 1: Read the following words out loud: Anxious, Afraid, Overwhelmed, Fragile, Depressed, Frustrated, Angry, Ashamed, Alone, Lonely, Exhausted, Numb.
STEP 2: Pick one of these words that most captures what you're feeling when you're greatly stressed and then focus on it.
STEP 3: Imagine feeling this feeling at its worst.
STEP 4: What does this feeling make you want to impulsively do?
STEP 5: Imagine saying what you want to do to a person who

loves you, and picture them smiling with love and compassion and saying back to you, "I understand."

STEP 6: Imagine feeling their love taking some of the pain away.

STEP 7: Imagine them asking you, "What would be a better thing to do?"

EXERCISE 3: TRAVELING THROUGH THE 12 PHASES EMOTIONAL ALGORITHM

Those who cannot remember the past are condemned to repeat it.

—GEORGE SANTAYANA

Take a good look at the quote above. Another way to say it would be, those who repress feelings during and after a trauma in order to survive are condemned to be terrorized by the past until they come to terms with and *move past* the past.

Once again, the 12 Phases Emotional Algorithm introduced in chapter 4 describes the process that leads to PTSD and the healing journey that follows. As a reminder, the pathway to PTSD looks like this:

Trauma → Horror → Terror → Fragile → Overriding Panic → Suppressed Thoughts → Repressed Feelings → Focus and Function → Danger Has Passed → PTSD → Disabled or Recovered → Healed

This 12 Phases Emotional Algorithm is a powerful key to recovery. When you empathetically revisit these phases one at a time and fully confront your feelings and thoughts at each, the process can help you heal.

The following exercise allows you to start at the point of trauma and empathically walk your earlier traumatized self through the process and back to the present. You can do this exercise repeatedly, and each time you will discover new insights that help you move further along your healing journey.

A quick word of caution about this exercise: revisiting traumatic memories can be a frightening, upsetting, and triggering experience that may bring up strong emotions, thoughts, and feelings. It may be best to do this next exercise with a therapist, particularly a Somatic Experiencing therapist. In fact, you might write down the list of the twelve phases above, share them with that therapist, and explain that they track fairly accurately with what you went through (or modify them to fit your experience even better). Then ask if the therapist would be able and willing to help you move through the phases.

You can also do this 12 Phases Emotional Algorithm exercise as a group. If you go this route, the moderator should lead the group on the path to and through PTSD and then on to healing. Again, if at any time during this exercise you become too overwhelmed or upset, do not continue. Instead, work with your therapist to create a plan for safely remembering and processing the trauma.

You can certainly try this exercise on your own, but do not hesitate to stop if it begins to increase your distress; you have not failed if you choose the therapist route. Remember, part of what made these phases so distressing was that you had to suppress and repress them in the first place, and that you faced them alone.

To do this exercise, set aside time when you won't be disturbed. Sit still and quiet your mind and body. Close your eyes. When you feel calm and ready, revisit each phase in the 12 Phases Emotional Algorithm below.

TRAUMA. Think back to the traumatizing event or events that created a fight, flight, or freeze response in your mind and body when it occurred. As you recall the event(s), make sure that you keep breathing. If you notice your heartbeat or breathing increasing, pause and focus on your breath before continuing to remember the trauma. Remind yourself that you survived and be compassionate toward your former self who was so upset at the time.

HORROR. Remember what it was like to feel the utter horror of the event(s). Allow yourself to experience any feelings of horror that you were unable to feel at the time because you had to keep going.

Remember to pause if you feel yourself becoming triggered by memories of this horror. If this happens take a few moments to look around and take in your environment. Look for five things you can see (for example: a window, a table, a pen). Think about what you feel (your shirt, your legs, the armrest of your chair), smell (the scent of rain), hear (traffic outside), and taste (the flavor of toothpaste). This will ground you in the present moment.

TERROR. Allow yourself to feel the terror you felt as your survival mechanisms (fight/flight/freeze) kicked in. Remember that we are meant to feel fear when we perceive danger. It is totally natural. Feel empathy for your earlier self who felt so afraid (and still feels afraid). With complete compassion and understanding, tell your former self (and your present self) that it is okay to feel afraid and that you are not alone.

FRAGILE. Lean into the fragility you felt and continue to feel following your trauma. Feel unconditional love, acceptance, and understanding for your earlier self who struggled to hold it together. Remind yourself that you are safe and secure right now, and that what was once shattered can be repaired.

OVERRIDING PANIC. Remember how it felt to override a panic response when you saw so many others in need and hurting, while you felt helpless and powerless. Remember being totally overwhelmed with feelings and emotions. Be gentle with yourself and try not to judge the way you reacted or wanted to react.

SUPPRESSED THOUGHTS. Remember the sheer exhaustion of trying to push aside everything you thought or were thinking. Feel empathy for your former self who had to bypass thoughts of guilt, shame, blame, and self-loathing to survive. Realize that these thoughts are normal to have, and that they don't make you a weak or shameful person. The thought really isn't the deed.

REPRESSED FEELINGS. To survive a trauma you pushed your feelings down so they would not bubble up into your conscious mind. Now other behaviors may have erupted due to this avoidance. What feelings are your coping behaviors (such as drinking, overeating, irritability) covering up? Spend time with every feeling that comes to mind. Acknowledge them fully and allow them to be felt.

FOCUS AND FUNCTION. Remember how it felt to put your own needs aside and rise to the occasion. You may recall the adrenaline rush you felt that helped you keep on going day after day, even as you knew something wasn't quite right deep inside. Focus on what it was like to put that assault to your inner well-being on the back burner. What did you neglect so you could help patients? What would you like to do for yourself now that you have some time to stop and reflect?

DANGER HAS PASSED. The horror and terror you experienced taunt you, and your new normal is a feeling in your body telling you that you must always be alert—especially when you revisit the place where the trauma occurred (most likely your workplace). How does this impact you today? What about your workplace triggers or unsettles you? Work to accept that while your work environment may not be as safe as you previously thought, this does not have to paralyze you or prevent you from living a full life.

PTSD. Immerse yourself in the pain of living with your trauma. Which routines and protective behaviors allow you to function in the world? How do they protect you? What would you do if you were not impacted by post-traumatic stress?

DISABLED OR RECOVERED. Can you label the emotions that come up again and again and make you feel stuck? These are the ones that must be fully felt before you can fully recover. With complete compassion, commit yourself to giving your feelings the space to exist. Allow them to be felt and shared, and notice how their power begins to fade.

HEALED. Finally, experiencing the emotions you pushed away to survive will drain the abscess and enable you to heal. Keep telling yourself that healing is possible and that you can once again feel peace and joy.

Post-traumatic stress not infrequently leads to post-traumatic growth. To put it simply, sometimes people not only heal but experience positive changes that occur after struggling through a trauma. You may find meaning in past events, deepened camaraderie, greater resilience, an understanding of what really matters, less worry over the "small stuff," and a liberating awareness of life's fragility, which empowers you to take life by the horns. Even if you are not there yet, you can look forward to the day when you notice the impact of post-traumatic growth in your life.

COGNITIVE BEHAVIORAL THERAPY

One of the most common treatment options for PTSD is Cognitive Behavioral Therapy (CBT). This type of psychotherapy has been shown to be effective for treating PTSD in the short and long term.[1] As you already know, PTSD creates patterns of thinking that lead to a cycle of anxiety, helplessness, and self-destructive behaviors. CBT breaks those vicious cycles and replaces them with a cycle of resilience and healing. As its name implies, CBT does this by addressing the patient's thinking (their cognition) and acting (their behaviors).

CBT harnesses and addresses the power of our thoughts, feelings, and actions. Normally our thoughts create healthy feedback loops. For example, you might think, *I've always wanted to learn to cook for my family. I think I will try to make a simple recipe tonight.* This thought inspires you to look up ingredients and try your hand at making a meal. When you accomplish a simple meal, you might decide to try a more complicated dish, and so forth.

PTSD creates feedback loops too—negative ones. People sometimes think overgeneralizing thoughts, catastrophizing thoughts, always/never thoughts, and so on. After COVID-19 you might start thinking thoughts such as, *I'm at fault for not saving my patient's life; I feel guilty for the death of my coworker. Did I do enough? Should I have intervened sooner?; I am ashamed that I feel numb about all this death. I don't feel anything anymore; I must not be very strong since I'm having all these feelings.*

The goal of CBT is to stop negative thought cycles by identifying the toxic thoughts, challenging them, replacing them with thoughts that make better sense and that point your life in a positive direction, and taking the same approach with any unproductive behaviors in which you engage.

Here are the main elements of Cognitive Behavioral Therapy.

Variety of Tools

CBT provides tools to help you feel safe when the moment at hand becomes too painful or intense. You might learn to use self-talk to dismiss negative thoughts and replace them with positive messages. Or you may learn breathing techniques and muscle relaxation to help your body release tension.

Exposure Therapy

You will also learn to confront trauma and the triggers that bring you back to it. One approach is called exposure therapy. There are different ways to approach this, and your therapist can help you find the best technique for you. You may confront the trauma one trigger at a time and work your way up to the most disturbing memories. Or you may face the memory as a whole and stick with the vivid memories for a prolonged time, repeating the process until the painful memories begin to fade. Your therapist may also ask you to return to the place your trauma occurred.

Cognitive Restructuring

A third component of CBT is cognitive restructuring, or undoing false ideas surrounding your trauma. This process achieves several things. First, it disputes your concerns about safety by confronting distorted thoughts such as, *I am a terrible person because I didn't do more to help.* Second, it addresses the desire to shut out others, which leaves you alone, angry, and bitter. Finally, it addresses guilt, which is a huge stumbling block to recovery. Your therapist will help you dismantle false beliefs about your trauma such as, *I didn't do enough to prevent this from happening.*

Life Application

Finally, CBT helps you use your new skills to improve your life. Together you and your therapist will explore the issues you want to work on next, apply what you've learned to real-life circumstances, and deal with any new challenges.

EYE MOVEMENT DESENSITIZATION AND REPROCESSING

Eye Movement Desensitization and Reprocessing, also called EMDR, is another very effective and efficient form of psychotherapy for treating PTSD. EMDR incorporates some of the CBT steps with a system of eye movements. It is based on the theory that the eye movements or other bilateral stimulation to the brain such as musical tones (not the therapist's verbal instructions) can help your memories of trauma become "unstuck" so you can process them in a healthy way. Much like CBT, it helps patients confront and process their original trauma, including upsetting memories, feelings, and thoughts that disrupt their lives.

Here's how EMDR works:

- Your therapist will prompt you to recall a memory associated with your trauma, and to rate how severely the memory distresses you.
- The therapist will ask you to identify negative beliefs related to the event, such as, "I failed my patients," or "I'll never forget witnessing so much death."
- Next you will be asked to create a positive thought that you would like to replace your negative belief with, perhaps "I am a great nurse," or "I can handle tough situations."
- You will also be asked to identify what you consider your "safe place," where you can mentally visit following the session's conclusion.
- Then you will watch the therapist's finger or pen moving back and forth—or listen to musical tones that switch back and forth from your left to right ear—while you recall your trauma. You will do this for brief periods and then in between repetitions discuss the feelings that arise with your therapist.
- The session ends when your level of distress has decreased and you feel aligned with the positive belief that you came up with at the beginning of your session.
- You will close by visualizing your safe place.

DIALECTICAL BEHAVIOR THERAPY

Another adaptation of CBT is Dialectical Behavior Therapy (DBT), which was created by Marsha Linehan. This evidence-based treatment was once used primarily for people with borderline personality disorder, but now it is also used for people suffering from PTSD as well as other issues. The word *dialectical* in DBT refers to the concept of balancing opposites. Therapists specializing in DBT work with their patient to learn to hold two seemingly opposite perspectives at once to avoid all-or-nothing types of thinking.

DBT focuses on helping patients develop new skills and behaviors to improve their lives. There are four key skills:

Mindfulness

This is the foundation for the other skills taught in DBT. Patients learn to nonjudgmentally accept the present moment by observing, describing, and participating in what is happening right now.

Distress Tolerance

Patients learn to tolerate overwhelming, negative emotions instead of trying to escape from them. They are taught skills to quickly alleviate distress, temporarily distract themselves from unpleasant emotions, nurture themselves, relax, and accept the unpleasant situation for what it is.

Emotional Regulation

This skill enables patients to change unwanted, problematic, and intense emotions. They are taught to identify and label the unwanted emotions; identify any obstacles in the way of changing them; reduce vulnerability by planning coping mechanisms in advance; and manage extreme conditions so they can remain stable and alert while in crisis.

Interpersonal Effectiveness

Finally, patients learn to communicate with others in a way that is assertive, that maintains respect, and that strengthens relationships.

They practice skills to help them achieve their goals in specific situations (such as requesting that someone do something or being able to say no to someone) while still maintaining the relationship and their own self-respect.

Patients undergoing DBT participate in three therapeutic settings. They attend individual therapy sessions with a DBT-certified therapist. They meet with other patients for group therapy, where they learn behavioral skills through homework assignments and role-playing. Finally, they have access to 24–7 phone coaching.

SOMATIC EXPERIENCING THERAPY

CBT is a top-down mode of therapy, meaning that it works with the thinking brain. Somatic Experiencing (SE) therapy is a bottom-up approach, which means it works with the body first to deal with the symptoms of trauma.

Developed by Dr. Peter Levine, SE is based on more than forty years of research and observation. His approach focuses on releasing traumatic shock, which is essential to transforming PTSD and the wounds of trauma.

SE addresses the freeze response, one of our three survival responses (fight, flight, or freeze). As a reminder, when people are threatened by danger, and when fight or flight is not possible, people instinctively freeze to make themselves less of a target.

Here's the problem with freezing: the freeze response is time sensitive. It needs to run its course, and the energy that was being stored while freezing must be dispelled through shaking and trembling. In nature, following the freeze response, animals shake for a short period of time and then move on without any problems. They literally "shake it off" and dispel the energy of the traumatic event.

For humans, however, if the freeze phase does not run its

course—for example if you are being held down by an attacker or bound by duty to stay in a terrifying situation to care for your patients—the energy can remain trapped in the body. This sends a message that the body is still under threat, which can cause all sorts of mental, emotional, and physical problems.

How Somatic Experiencing Works

Somatic Experience helps patients release their stored energy and turn off the threat alarm that can cause severe dissociation and dysregulation of the autonomic nervous system. In SE sessions you won't be asked to focus on the particulars of the traumatic event. Instead you will explore the body sensations linked to the feelings around the event. Your therapist will frequently check in with you about your somatic sensations such as tightness or heaviness.

Resourcing is a practice used in SE. It helps you develop strategies to consciously impact the nervous system in a healthy and nurturing way, rather than a dysfunctional way. A resource is anything you can access to create a sense of calm and safety. It could be thinking of a beautiful sunset or a mountain vista, or recalling a favorite memory.

You will move slowly in your sessions. Your therapist will gradually help you revisit the trauma and its associated sensations. This is called *titration*. This process slows the "too fast, too soon" nature of the trauma so you can handle it.

Another practice your therapist will use is called *pendulation*— moving gently between accessing internal sensations and traumatic memories. This helps your nervous system get used to moving between alertness and calm without getting stuck.

To learn more about Somatic Experiencing, you can read Dr. Levine's bestselling book *Waking the Tiger: Healing Trauma*. In the meantime, here are exercises inspired by Dr. Levine's work.

Dr. Levine's Voo Breathing Exercise

One of Dr. Levine's popular techniques is his Voo Exercise, which can help calm your nervous system and stimulate the vagus nerve. This is the cranial nerve that runs from the neck to the abdomen and controls the parasympathetic ("rest and digest") nervous system responses. To try the exercise, follow the steps below.

1. Take time to quiet yourself so you feel calm and safe, and spend a few moments noticing your breath.
2. Breathe in deeply through your nose. When you do this make sure you breathe into your belly (not into your chest).
3. Breath out and make a "voo" sound on your exhale. Try to imitate the sound of a foghorn.
4. When you run out of breath, breathe in deeply again. Do the exercise three to five times and see if you feel settled.

Dr. Levine's Self-Hold Exercise

Our bodies are the containers of our thoughts and emotions. People with trauma in their histories may have trouble feeling their boundaries. They often feel scattered all over the place. This simple exercise helps you connect to your boundaries and your container. Here's what to do:

1. Take your right hand and place it underneath your left arm on the side of your heart.
2. Take your left hand and place it on the outside of the right arm.
3. Hold this position for several minutes until you notice a settling come over you.
4. Repeat anytime you feel overwhelmed or stressed.

You can watch a video of Peter demonstrating this exercise, along

with a few other useful exercises, by visiting this site: https://www
.nicabm.com/trauma-two-simple-techniques-that-can-help-trauma
-patients-feel-safe/.

TAPPING THERAPY

Two of the most popular forms of Tapping Therapy are the Emotional
Freedom Technique and Field Thought Therapy. These holistic techniques are derived from Eastern medicine philosophies and aim to
balance the body's energy system.

The premise behind tapping is that the negative emotions caused
by trauma disrupt the body's energy flow. Tapping while addressing
negative memories and emotions brings the body back into balance.

Here's an overview of a tapping exercise: First, recall a disturbing
thought, emotion, fear, or memory. As you do this, tap on various
meridian points on the body (such as the top of the head, the collar-
bone, etc.). By tapping on these points, you assist your body's energy in
flowing freely. Your therapist can show you the correct tapping technique and direct you on where to tap. After every round of tapping,
your therapist will ask you questions about whether your feelings are
changing.

To learn more about tapping you can read *The Tapping Solution*
by Nick Ortner. You can also check out the Tapping with Brad exercises on YouTube by visiting https://www.youtube.com/c/tapwithbrad
/featured.

MEDICATION: TO TAKE OR NOT TO TAKE?

In addition to therapeutic approaches, your healthcare provider may
suggest medication as another treatment option. Medicine may not

be the right choice for everyone, but for some, prescription drugs are a good option for treating the symptoms of PTSD.

There are many pros of taking medication. It can:

- nip a crisis in the bud before things spiral out of control;
- provide a stopgap until you can be seen by a therapist;
- treat not only PTSD but other coexisting disorders such as depression; and
- turn your life around by enabling you to get plenty of sleep, go to work, maintain healthy relationships, and find joy in your life again.

Of course, there are downsides to medications as well. They can be habit-forming, they can cause side effects, and once your brain adapts to a drug it can sometimes stop being as effective.

Before taking a new prescription drug, work with your doctor to decide if it is the right medication for you. Here are questions we often coach our patients to ask, but it is important to remember to ask them ourselves as patients.

- What does this medication do?
- How long does it take for this drug to work?
- How long will I need to take this drug?
- What are the side effects? Could this drug make me suicidal? (Certain medications for preventing depression can raise your risk of having suicidal thoughts or feelings.)
- Will this medication cause dependency?
- What are the withdrawal effects of taking this drug?
- Can I safely take this drug with the other medications and/or supplements I take?
- Are there certain foods or beverages that interact with this drug?
- (If pregnant) Will this drug be safe for my unborn baby?

When you and your doctor have decided on the best medication for you, be mindful of taking the correct dosage at the right time each day. Set an alarm on your phone to remind you if you cannot remember to take your medication, or train yourself to do it in tandem with another daily habit, such as brushing your teeth.

Pay close attention to your body's response when taking your new medication. If you start experiencing serious side effects either mentally (such as confusion, aggressive impulses, extreme restlessness, or suicidal feelings) or physically (such as severe nausea or vomiting, heart palpitations, fainting, or difficulty breathing), contact your doctor immediately. Finally, never stop taking a medication without talking to your doctor. Abruptly stopping medication can cause dangerous withdrawal symptoms. You may need to be weaned off slowly.

Yes, as a healthcare worker, you most definitely know this stuff already. But remember that these directions apply for all patients, even those who are healthcare professionals themselves. Set a great example to your patients and listen to your own advice!

As you can see, many good treatment options for PTSD exist, and now you also have a few exercises to help you begin a healing journey. In chapter 6 we will cover the process of finding a therapist and look at other advice you can implement immediately to facilitate your healing.

HELP YOURSELF:

What You Can Do to Start Healing Today

DR. MARK GOULSTON

Living with the symptoms of PTSD can make you feel like your life is spinning out of control, but there is a lot that you can do right now to start the healing process. Following these best practices will not instantaneously change your life, but they will set in motion the steps necessary for reclaiming your life bit by bit, and eventually you will feel their impact.

FIND A GOOD THERAPIST

Working with a skilled therapist is an important part of recovery. There is a stigma in healthcare around seeking therapy, but maybe it's time to ask yourself, "How well am I handling this on my own? When I rush to reassure the world and myself that I'm fine, am I really? What are some of the unhealthy habits—overeating, drinking too much, self-medicating, sleeping excessively—I've developed that I tell myself I'm in control of but I'm really not?"

If your personal assessment comes back as, "Who am I kidding, I'm not handling this," therapy can be a beneficial addition to your life. I urge you to be open to what it can do for you. At the end of the day your good health is one of the most important things in your life, and mental health certainly plays a role in your overall wellness.

And don't worry or be embarrassed. More of your fellow health-care providers than you can imagine would come up with the same answers that they're not doing so well.

How do you find a good therapist? There's no one right way to find a good match, but these guidelines can help. You may want to begin by asking for a referral from your primary care doctor. But you can also check with other people you trust, such as your minister, priest, or rabbi, trustworthy friends or relatives, a local support group for individuals with PTSD, or your HR department at work.

Once you have a prospective therapist in mind, check out their training and experience. Ideally, your therapist will have a master's degree or doctorate, and will be skilled and experienced in treating PTSD.

Meet with your potential therapist and ask them lots of questions. Here are a few to begin with:

- *What approaches do you use, and do you feel that they will be right for me?* Therapists use various approaches to treat PTSD, some of which have been described in this book. Ask them their thoughts on the kinds of therapy that will work best for you.
- *From your point of view, what is PTSD, what do you think causes it, and what needs to happen for a person to get better or recover from it?* The reason to ask this is to see if what they say *makes sense, feels like it would work*, and actually seems *doable by and with you*. If what they say makes sense, feels right, and

seems doable, it will increase your confidence and hope that it could work.

- *How do you feel about medication?* Ideally, you will both have similar philosophies about medication.
- *When can we meet?* Find out what their session schedule is like. The more your schedules line up, the easier it will be to meet.
- *How long do you think my therapy will last?* Every patient is different, and your therapist cannot fully predict how many sessions you will need, but they should be able to give you an idea as to whether your treatment should be short-term or long-term.
- *How much will therapy cost?* Your therapist should be able to check your insurance information and give you an estimate of your out-of-pocket costs. They can also tell you whether they accept payments from your insurer or whether you will need to pay now and be reimbursed by your insurer.
- *Are you available in an emergency?* Therapists should be reachable if you have a true emergency. Find out if they will take calls outside office hours.

After you find a good therapist with whom you can build rapport and trust, stick to your sessions. Some appointments may feel easy while others may be excruciatingly painful. You might feel on top of the world one day and hopelessly helpless the next. Setbacks are a normal part of the process. What's important is that you keep showing up. Eventually you will be able to look back and see how far you have come.

FORM YOUR FIRE TEAM

Remember the importance of reflecting on the traumatic events you and your colleagues experienced together. Think of the comfort you feel when you have a chance to share, vent, and debrief with your teammates during or after a rough shift. They are the only ones who can truly understand what you have been through, because they also went through it. You can lean on one another for strength and support as you deal with the fallout of being on the front lines of COVID-19.

If your organization has not already formed a support group for its employees, consider starting a weekly informal meeting in which you and your coworkers can gather and talk about what you are going through. You may be surprised to find that others have been suffering as well. This not only gives you a community in which to share about your mental and emotional struggles (and yes, your triumphs too!), but it also will help remove the stigma surrounding mental illness in the healthcare community. Now it is more important than ever that healthcare providers be empowered to shine a light on their pain and get the help they need.

FACE YOUR SUBSTANCE ABUSE ISSUES (IF YOU HAVE ANY)

There's a big difference between enjoying a glass of wine to unwind after work and developing a dependency or addiction on alcohol or other substances. It's important to hold yourself accountable if you are self-medicating with drugs and drinks. Look out for warning signs like these:

- You minimize or rationalize your excessive use of substances.
- You have tried (unsuccessfully) to cut back on drinking or drug use.
- Loved ones have commented on or expressed concern over your use of alcohol or drugs.

- You feel shame about how much you drink or how often you use drugs.
- You have trouble staying fully present because you're thinking of when you can have your next drink or take another dose of your drug of choice.
- You need a drink to get through the day.

The problem with using substances to cope with PTSD is that the relief you feel is temporary and doesn't fix the root of the problem. Further, the helplessness you feel because of PTSD is exacerbated by the helplessness of substance dependency or addiction. Substance abuse also creates new problems on top of your existing struggles.

If you know or suspect you have a problem with alcohol or drug abuse, talk to your therapist. They can help you make important decisions about your treatment and tailor a protocol that supports all your needs.

LEARN THE BASICS OF ANGER MANAGEMENT

Anger, which is a normal human emotion, can reach unhealthy levels when a person has PTSD or has faced trauma. When it spirals out of control, it can harm you and your loved ones.

If your anger makes you physically violent or so verbally aggressive that you frighten yourself or others, you need to seek professional help immediately. Even if your anger has not reached this level, it is a good idea to tell your therapist you are having anger issues and begin working to conquer this.

Here are a few guidelines for preventing uncontrolled outbursts when your anger is not so severe as to be a threat to yourself or others.

When Anger Hits, Take Stock of What's Really Going On

This is a great way to get control of your emotions (not just anger) and impulses.

- Notice where you feel tension and anger in your body. Are you clenching your teeth? Is there a knot in your stomach?
- Answer the question, "What does this anger make me want to do?" The answer might be to tell your coworker to shut up or to scream at the next person you see.
- Imagine what would happen if you actually do the thing you impulsively want to do. Mentally review all possible outcomes.
- Ask yourself, "What is a better thing to do instead?"
- Finish the sentence, "If I do this strategy (instead of what I feel like doing), the benefits will be _____."

Take a Time-Out

When anger surges, whenever possible cool down by leaving the scene. Excuse yourself if you are with someone else, and go for a quick walk or at least head to the restroom until you can control your temper.

Use "I" Messages

Instead of focusing on another person's faults in an angry rant, turn your focus to how you feel. This can head off a fight and transform it into a respectful conversation. Rather than telling your partner, "You never ask me for my input. You are selfish and do exactly what you want to do every time!" you could use "I" messages and try saying, "When you don't ask me to weigh in before you make important decisions, I feel like my needs are unimportant to you. It makes me feel sad and I am more hesitant to speak up every time it happens." You may notice that unlike the first sentence, which felt like an accusation, the second version gives insight to your true feelings and does not blame the other person.

Get Some Exercise

We'll touch on this later in this chapter, but exercise is a great way to get out angry energy. When you feel your anger surging, go for a run, do aerobic exercise, or tackle heavy-duty yard work or house-cleaning. When you're done you will have accomplished something productive while working off your adrenaline rush.

GET RID OF TOXIC PEOPLE IN YOUR LIFE

This is a great time to let go of anyone who does not want the best for you. Doing this may be difficult in the moment, but in the long run you'll be far better off surrounding yourself with a supportive network of people who truly want you to thrive. You can either make a clean break with this toxic person (or people) or gradually phase them out of your life.

If you cannot completely separate because the toxic person is a family member or someone you see every day, such as a boss or coworker, set healthy boundaries. For example, tell your sister that you can only visit (or Skype or Zoom in the age of the coronavirus) once a month instead of weekly. If someone at work is the problem, do your best to reduce your contact with that person—maybe ask to be reassigned to a new team or try to work a different shift. If it is impossible to separate yourself entirely, your therapist can give you pointers on healthy ways to cope.

HANDLE THE DEMANDS OF WORK

Since most people need to work for a living, you will likely need to continue working while dealing with the trauma of COVID-19. Unfortunately for healthcare workers, your work environment played a major role in your trauma in the first place. Your fears and memories are no doubt still fresh. Therefore, be gentle with yourself in the workplace. Yes, you have important work to do, but you can incorporate small routines and tools that help you get through each day, including the rough ones. Here are a few things that can be in your wellness toolbox.

Instant Relaxation Techniques

Keep a list of quick and simple ways you can relieve tension at work, and do one or two of the techniques each time you take a break. Take a sixty-second stretching session. Close your eyes and breathe deeply for two minutes. Do a brief grounding exercise by noticing five things that you can see, smell, taste, touch, and hear. Give yourself a quick shoulder massage.

Something That Makes You Laugh

Humor is a great way to alleviate stress. Tape a clip of a funny cartoon to your work area or carry a small notebook with jokes that make you laugh every time you read them.

Calming Affirmations

Written positive statements can give you a lift when you feel yourself sinking, and if self-talk is not for you, imagine a supportive other saying these to you in your mind's eye. A few examples:

I am great at my job, and my training and skills are empowering.
I feel energized and ready for anything the day has in store for me.
I accept myself as I am. I am enough.
I am safe in this moment.

Anchors

Carry a small reminder of what you love about your life. It might be a photo of your kids or pet, or a small rock you picked up on a scenic nature hike. Think of the gratitude you feel for your life whenever you look at this token.

GET YOUR NUTRITION IN ORDER

When you are dealing with PTSD, healthy habits often take a back-seat. Instead of cooking nutrient-rich meals, you are more likely to rely on takeout or microwaved dinners. You're also more likely to crave carb-heavy comfort foods that provide a boost of serotonin but often cause unhealthy blood sugar levels.

Don't waste a moment feeling guilty over past or current bad eating habits. But do take these positive steps to giving your body the fuel it needs to feel your best.

Start Making Healthy Substitutions Today

You don't have to transform your habits overnight, but you can swap in healthy choices. Replace a serving of chips with a piece of fruit. Cook chicken breasts for dinner instead of opting for that frozen burrito. Pack a healthy homemade lunch instead of eating pizza in the work cafeteria. Cut down on sodas and replace them with glasses of filtered water. These small changes will add up quickly.

Pop a Vitamin

A multivitamin can help ensure you are getting vitamins and minerals essential for health. You might also include a fish oil supplement, which provides omega-3 fatty acids that play a role in brain and heart health.

Avoid Fad Diets

Fad diets may help you drop excess weight quickly, but they are lots of work and most people find they are too hard to stick to. You don't need anything in your life that puts you in an "I failed again" mindset. Stick to a slow and steady approach to weight loss through sensible food choices and exercise.

GET PLENTY OF EXERCISE

Headaches, backaches, and other pain related to tension in the body can occur after enduring a trauma. Exercise can help you release some of the "frozen" tension you may be carrying around. It also releases endorphins, the feel-good chemical, while giving yourself a great distraction from stress and worry.

The most important part of exercise is consistency, so choose fitness activities you enjoy. These could be going for a daily walk around your neighborhood, streaming workout videos, joining a virtual dance class, or going for a light jog. Don't forget daily stretching as well, to keep your muscles limber. Aim for thirty minutes of activities at least three times a week, and you will be well on your way to becoming not only physically healthier but emotionally healthier.

If you are not used to exercising, remember to take things slow; you are less likely to injure yourself and more likely to stick with your program. Another word of caution: if exercising puts you at risk of hyperventilation or panic attacks, talk to your therapist about techniques to help manage or prevent them, such as breathing exercises.

MEDITATE

A simple meditation routine can help you maintain a more relaxed state overall and help you manage anxiety or other symptoms of PTSD. If you are new to meditation, follow this mindfulness-based meditation routine to relax and become present.

- Close your eyes and begin slowly breathing in and out through your nose.
- As you do this, take note of the world around you. You may notice the sounds outside or sensations in your own body.
- Allow your emotions and thoughts to rise and flow through you naturally. Do your best to avoid judging them as they pass by. Simply let them be.
- If a particular thought or feeling arises during your meditation, acknowledge it gently (again, no judging) and release it. For example, you might feel afraid and think, *I am frightened.* Stay with this feeling in the moment and then gently and peacefully let it go. What is left is often the quiet, and you can be present in the quiet when you let go of everything else.

Don't fret if you are unable to start off meditating for twenty or thirty minutes at a time. Most people find that they need to work their way up. Start by aiming for two minutes, and when you get comfortable with that amount of time, try five minutes, and so on.

PRACTICE GROUNDING

Like meditation, grounding is a great way to reduce anxiety. We have covered a few basic grounding practices already, but here is a more in-depth grounding exercise you can try. It is effective at helping you arrive in the here and now. Use it any time you feel carried away by anxious thoughts, feelings, or upsetting memories and flashbacks.

- Find a comfortable place to sit. A comfortable sofa or chair works best.

- Rest your hands on the arms of the chair or, if the chair has no arms, place them on your legs. Feel the fabric of the chair or your clothing. Notice its color and texture.
- Next, bring your awareness to your body. Stretch your neck from side to side. Relax your shoulders. Tense and relax your calves. Stomp your feet.
- Look around and notice the sights, sounds, and scents around you for a few moments.
- Name fifteen to twenty things you can see. For example, your phone, a lamp, a glass of water, or the carpet.
- As you keep looking around, remind yourself that "The flashback or emotion I felt is in the past. Right now, in this moment, I'm safe."

RELAX YOUR BODY

This progressive relaxation exercise can help you release tension all over the body as a way to manage daily stress.

- Start by either lying down or sitting in a chair. Keep your feet slightly apart and place your arms by your sides, palms facing up. Close your eyes.
- Slowly and evenly breathe in and out as you silently count to twenty.
- Now, starting with your feet, contract the muscles of your feet and toes while you slowly count to five. Then relax your feet and toes as you count to twenty.
- Follow the same steps for each muscle group as you progressively move up your body: ankles, calves, thighs, glutes, stomach, chest, hands, biceps, upper arms, shoulders, neck, and face.

VISUALIZE YOUR WAY TO A SAFER, HAPPIER STATE

This exercise uses the power of your mind to help you feel safe and calm. Practice this visualization or create a visualization centered around another safe space anytime you wish.

- Close your eyes and imagine that you are lying on a blanket in a field on a perfectly warm and sunny day. Nearby there are majestic trees and patches of colorful flowers. You can hear chirping birds and the quiet trickle of a woodland creek.
- Deepen the visualization to incorporate your senses. Hear the water running over stones and logs. Feel the sun warming your face. Feel the softness of the blanket juxtaposed with the grass tickling your fingers. Notice a woodchuck scamper by. Look up as a few puffy clouds drift above your head.
- When you feel relaxed and refreshed, slowly open your eyes and take in the light of the room. Look around and reorient yourself to the present moment and the real world. Breathe deeply and stretch. When you are ready, go about your day.

NOTICE THE SIMPLE PLEASURES AROUND YOU

PTSD can make the world seem terribly dangerous, with threats lurking around every corner. That's why it is important to stay immersed in the joys of life. Focusing on fun, simple pleasures is a good way to promote healing and enjoy your life in the process.

Get Lost in a Good Book

Don't just read a few pages before bedtime. Really allow yourself to indulge. Set aside thirty minutes after work or in the morning before starting your day to escape into a captivating story.

Cook a Delicious Meal

Cooking can be a fun and enjoyable experience, even for novices. Instead of opting for takeout, look up a simple new recipe and give it a try. You get to enjoy a homecooked meal while gaining confidence from trying something new.

Take a Walk

Even if it is only five minutes long, commit to taking a walk every day. If nothing else circle the block or walk to the end of your driveway. Chances are, by the time those five minutes are up, you will want to keep going. Take in the sights around you and you will notice the gifts of nature—a busy squirrel, drifting clouds, your neighbor's flower beds.

Find a Creative Outlet

Think gardening, playing a musical instrument, putting together a puzzle, or even coloring in an adult coloring book.

Hit the Pause Button

If you tend to go-go-go without ever taking a break, do the opposite by making time for mandatory relaxation. Walk to a park and people watch. Draw a bubble bath. Sit on your porch and enjoy a glass of lemonade.

BRIGHTEN SOMEONE'S DAY

PTSD can create a layer of self-involvement that cloisters you from regular social interactions that keep you healthy. Even if it feels strange, go out of your way to interact with strangers each day. Smile at passersby. Ask if you may pet a neighbor's dog. Have a friendly chat with someone living on your block. Go over to a homeless person(s), say hello, tell them your name, and ask them theirs (they do have names). Always carry a bag of healthy snacks with you to give away, saying, "Here [their name], I hope this helps." This is a great reminder that you care about others. It will also make you feel good for doing something that demonstrates some of your kindness to the world *and* you.

CONSIDER GETTING AN ANIMAL COMPANION

If you don't already have a pet, consider adopting a furry friend. Cats, dogs, and other domestic animals can be so helpful to people going through crises. If you don't want to commit to ownership right now (after all, it's a big responsibility), ask a friend or family member if they will allow their pet to visit you for a weekend of snuggles and fun. You can also consider fostering or volunteering for a rescue organization.

And if you already have an animal companion, don't forget that they are a source of endless love and affection. Embrace and enjoy caring for a creature who loves and needs you. Giving of yourself will reward you as much as it does them.

TRY NEW THINGS

PTSD can cause you to shy away from doing new things that might challenge you. It keeps you alert and ready to react to any new threat, so you may prefer to maintain the status quo by sticking to your existing routines and habits. But exploring new relationships, activities, and interests is an important part of a healthy lifestyle.

Brainstorm new things you would like to bring into your life. These might be new skills such as coding, improv, martial arts, or learning a new language. Or perhaps you would like to start dating, or plan a road trip, or have another sort of new experience. You can take steps to make these a reality starting now. There is no shortage of adventures you can have (or look forward to having in the future when the pandemic is over). What matters is remaining open to doing new things in the first place.

TALK ABOUT THE TRAUMA

Remember the Six *H*s: having horror heard helps heal hurt. This is a powerful truth at the foundation of healing, so share your feelings about your trauma with trusted close friends and family members. You will feel less alone and your upsetting feelings will become less awful. Panic can lessen into just fear. Anger can dissipate until you just feel frustrated and annoyed.

But keep in mind that you don't have to describe every excruciating detail of your trauma or relive memories that frighten you. Focus on the parts you are comfortable remembering. Maybe you can describe the before and after events instead of the scariest moments. And remember that you can also confide in your coworkers who are part of your fire team—they know better than anyone exactly what you have been through and are likely also dealing with the aftermath.

Remember that it may be hard for people to hear your feelings without wanting to fix your problems or tell you that "it will all be okay because you're strong." To circumvent these well-meaning but ultimately unhelpful responses, ask the other person to simply listen to you.

One tactic that may help the other person be there with you in the way you need them to be is showing *them* empathy regarding *their* discomfort. If you do that, you might ironically cause both of you to feel better by taking care of someone else.

You can do this by smiling at them and saying, "That's okay. If I were you, I wouldn't know what to say either, and I'd also want to rush to make it better. But what will help me more is you just letting me get my feelings out without you feeling pressure to do or say anything. Just that will help me feel better and calmer, and it sure beats talking to myself."

After surviving a trauma that shakes your foundations, you may feel that life as you knew it is gone forever. That is simply not true. Though you may never forget your experiences around COVID-19, you absolutely can reclaim your life and begin to find peace, joy, and happiness again. You now have information on many of the treatments and tools that can help you transform from a person who copes to a person who heals. This may not always be an easy journey, but it is absolutely one worth making. Living through hard times makes us stronger in many ways. We can look back and see that we survived something that we didn't think we could. Overcoming challenges also increases our capacity for gratitude. We are more able to savor the small joys in life—of which there are many.

Watch for signs that you are making progress—they will likely show up when you least expect them. One day you will wake up and notice that you are looking forward to the day ahead. Another time you will realize you just navigated a difficult conversation without getting overwhelmed or angry. Your sense of optimism will show up one day out of the blue. Hold tight to these moments when you are struggling, and feel tremendous gratitude for them when they grace you on the good days. And when the day comes that you feel more like yourself than you have in ages, you will realize just how far you have come.

CHAPTER 7

A CALL TO ACTION: LEADING THROUGH THE PANDEMIC—AND BEYOND

DR. DIANA HENDEL

IT IS UNDENIABLE

Healthcare professionals are among the most resilient, grittiest, and strongest people in our society, and their behaviors often reflect a deeply felt sense of purpose and meaning. For many, work is a *calling*. They know the joy of bringing new life into the world. The joy of saving or healing those injured or ill. And, they know the feeling of despair when healing is not possible.

Under normal circumstances the environment they work in is complicated and complex. Because there are lots of hand-offs and moving parts in a healthcare organization's operation, collaboration and coordination are paramount to ensuring the best possible outcomes. A highly functioning operation fosters a profound spirit of camaraderie, teamwork, and unity—and the kind of fulfillment that comes from being part of something much larger than oneself and from accomplishing things that cannot be done by one person alone. But the stakes are extraordinarily high. If not done well, the consequences can be disastrous, deadly even, for patients. And, in the face of COVID-19, for healthcare workers as well.

Healthcare workers are accustomed to high stress, frequent challenges, changing circumstances, and the unpredictability that comes with caring for human beings. They thrive in these conditions. They are used to dealing with things that cannot be entirely controlled. Like a heavy workload. Like implementing a new electronic health record. Like unannounced regulatory inspections. Like sudden changes in a patient's clinical condition. They've been "tried and tested" through intense training and through their lived experiences. For many, there is little they haven't seen in the healthcare arena. Until now.

Laypeople think that healthcare professionals are accustomed to death—and, yes, death does loom large on the front lines, and the possibility of it is never far from mind. For that reason, policies and procedures underscore the "on guard" nature of their workplaces and reflect the importance of the work they do to save lives and prevent death. Every process is outlined meticulously and every detail is attended to so that errors are reduced, adverse reactions are quickly identified, and death is minimized.

For most clinicians and caregivers, though, death does not occur as frequently as depicted in a TV drama or medical soap opera. I don't know a healthcare professional who doesn't remember every single death that has occurred on their watch, and many report that they felt responsible in some way or another. This sense of responsibility is embedded in our healthcare culture, expected by society, and wholeheartedly accepted by all those who have taken a sacred oath.

And aren't we glad to know this is how our clinicians and caregivers approach their professions? Who wouldn't want their surgeon or labor-and-delivery nurse or respiratory care therapist or pharmacist to feel responsible when they perform their patient-care duties? And let's never forget that this feeling of responsibility also extends to many others on the team who serve in ancillary and supportive roles: housekeepers, facilities engineers, administrators, sterile processing personnel, and security guards are just a few examples of the thousands of roles that exist within our healthcare facilities and systems. Whether their work is performed behind the scenes or they interact directly with patients, they are vitally important in safeguarding the health and well-being of patients, visitors, and their coworkers.

It's long been known that a healthcare professional's greatest strengths—dedication, commitment, and sense of responsibility—can also lead to compassion fatigue, overworking, and burnout, even under the best of circumstances. But the stress and pressure of COVID-19, which is persistent and relentless, frequently overwhelming, and ostensibly never ending, could stretch anyone to the near breaking point.

IT IS UNDERSTANDABLE

The COVID-19 pandemic presents a trifecta of trauma and turmoil and tragedy that threatens the physical and emotional well-being of the heroes charged with caring for others.

Healthcare facilities in our society have long been considered safe havens, but this pandemic has shattered that assumption of safety. Patients are usually brought to a hospital or clinic for care for an injury or illness acquired on the outside. And, to be sure, that happened following the COVID-19 outbreak, as patients began arriving in droves. But for those healthcare workers on the inside, it also created great risk of contracting an unpredictably lethal disease or of becoming an asymptomatic vector and transmitting it to others.

With limited or nonexistent PPE in the early days, the fear of becoming infected, or infecting others, was palpable. (And though healthcare workers have shown ingenuity in adapting to shortages in PPE [and ventilators and medications and supplies!], as of this writing, this fear still exists, as scarcity remains commonplace in many healthcare facilities.) Added to that, there was (and is) anxiety from not being able to guarantee the safety from infection for their other, non-COVID-19 patients. Though elective procedures had initially come to a screeching halt, patients with high-risk births, cardiac or neurological emergencies, and life-threatening cancers are still very much in need of care. And, on top of all that, healthcare workers worry about the danger of infecting their own family members when they return home from a long shift, which has forced many to make the hard choice of living separately to protect them.

Then there are the harrowing reports of patients gasping helplessly for breath in the last moments of their life. Since they must be physically separated from their loved ones, caregivers hold up iPads to virtually connect them, all the while holding the patient's hand with their gloved one. Though powerless to stop their patient from dying, they remain bedside, not shying away from duty. Simultaneously, they feel both sadness and honor—sadness of another senseless death and honor at being able to be with them in their last moments, knowing that they didn't die alone.

These end-of-life circumstances, which sometimes exceed ten-plus per day, are unnerving even for the steely minded. And knowing that their patients' bodies will be placed in a morgue that is overflowing—so much so that refrigerated trailers line their pathway as they arrive and depart each shift—only adds to their angst and stress. As if the constant physical reminders of this pandemic's seriousness—masking, shielding, gowning up, and temperature checks on arrival—were not already ever present.

Add to that the threat of personal financial insecurity at a time when they are working harder than ever, as healthcare organizations grapple with revenue shortfalls and increases in expenses, and rumors of layoffs or furloughs or salary cuts circulate ruthlessly.

The toll on our healthcare workforce extends into moral territory as well. Over time the shortages in supplies and resources and space have pushed many organizations to limits previously unimagined. Faced with scarcity, ethics, and triage, committees are forced to confront dilemmas about who gets care and who doesn't—who is too sickly to take valuable resources from someone else who is deemed savable—in short, who lives and who dies.

The environment our healthcare professionals work in now feels much less physically and psychologically safe than it did before COVID-19. And inarguably, it is.

Initially, the biological reactions of fight, flight, and freeze are to be expected in response to a trauma like COVID-19. But over time frustration, uncertainty, and sheer exhaustion understandably shift to intractable anger and despair. "It all seems so unnecessary!" they may scream silently. But in our stoic and stiff-upper-lip culture, feelings of fear and anxiety and grief are often shouldered solitarily, privately, and hidden behind a brave, public face of strength and resolve.

And remaining chronically in survival mode leads to the very real concern that PTSD may be inevitable for many on the front lines facing a ceaseless barrage—if they are unable to get the help they need and deserve.

IT MAY RESULT IN PTSD

I've been there: privately tortured but publicly showing a face of strength and resolve, after surviving and leading through the aftermath of a deadly trauma in my workplace. And the experience changed me as a person and as a leader.

Like many other healthcare professionals, I "grew up" in a

healthcare organization. For me that was a large medical center complex that for more than one hundred years had been a venerable, trusted fixture in the community. I'd arrived as a student and stayed on as a clinical pharmacy resident and then as a hospital management resident before becoming a permanent member of the staff. Over the next twenty years I was progressively promoted throughout the health system to bigger leadership roles with more and more responsibility. In early 2009, I became CEO of two large acute care, teaching hospitals—one focused on caring for adults and the other on the unique needs of children—that shared a campus in Long Beach, California.

Throughout my career I'd had numerous encounters with adversity and a lot of experience managing the unexpected—from operational mishaps to financial hardship to minor scandals, disasters, and PR nightmares. Our teams and I had also been well trained and seasoned in crisis management—after all, trauma was a big part of our business—but it was almost always *other* people's traumas we faced. People came to us for care; rarely had we been in a position of responding to our own internal trauma.

But one day early in my tenure as CEO, a man came to the main lobby of the hospital and shot the supervisor of the outpatient pharmacy several times at point-blank range. He then ran through to the other side of the hospital, where he shot the executive director of the pharmacy department before turning the gun on himself. All three died on site.

As anyone could well imagine, it was horrifying for those who witnessed the shootings and for all of us who responded to the scenes. But regardless of proximity or involvement, it was traumatic for everyone because the shooter was an insider—a staff member beloved by many and recently honored as our employee of the quarter—who had killed his bosses.

As an acute care provider, we couldn't close or stop caring for patients. We couldn't completely stop to regroup. We still had more than six hundred patients in-house who needed our care. Like the oft-cited business idiom, we had to continue flying the plane and repair it at the same time.

Since we had not gone through a trauma as severe or as emotionally wrenching as this before, many things happened in the aftermath that we had not anticipated or imagined were possible. And though we made mistakes, we also did a good job in many ways of managing the trauma. The structure of a familiar and well-practiced incident command system provided focus and direction, kept us aligned toward common goals, and helped to steady our emotions. Responding to the trauma revealed an amazing esprit de corps and exposed an extraordinary degree of connectedness and camaraderie. We developed newfound appreciation and respect for one another. Through our collective experience, our commitment to purpose and meaning was reinforced and we became more tightly bound together than we had been before.

But even though the event was over, its impact didn't end on the day of the shooting; for many, it had just begun. Those closest to the epicenter of the trauma were caught in a web of guilt, shame, blame—and fear. Guilt that we'd survived while our colleagues had not. Shame that the shooter had been one of us. Blame that we hadn't prevented it or stopped it. Or maybe that we'd caused it. And fear because there had been no prior signs from the shooter that hinted at the violence to come. Was there another among us capable of that as well? Some would torture themselves believing they'd missed a clue or were somehow complicit by complaining about management. We did a lot of second-guessing. Should there have been bullet-proof glass in the pharmacy? Should the security guards have been armed? Had our background checks failed us? Had the organization done enough to prevent it? Had the recent announcements about layoffs played a part?

But within a relatively short period of time, the organization rebounded, moved on, and grew stronger than it had been before. Our communication philosophies and practices, team-building and succession-planning activities, and decision-making processes were transformed as a direct result of our experience with the trauma. All of which, ultimately, made us better prepared to deal with future traumas (we came to realize that it was not a matter of if, but when). And to perform better in routine, everyday situations.

So why am I telling this story about a workplace shooting, a trauma that is both relatively rare and an extreme example?

I tell it because the effects of the COVID-19 pandemic are strikingly similar to what I experienced as an individual and what I observed as the leader of a traumatized organization.

I tell it because every day I am in contact with clinicians and leaders who tell me how COVID-19 has impacted them and others within their organizations. They describe being both in the crosshairs and in the crossfire as they share the enormous pressure, stress, and fear they are feeling.

I tell it because I, too, experienced many of the same feelings that my healthcare clients and colleagues are now experiencing as they struggle to manage the COVID-19 pandemic in their facilities and practices. The shock, the terror, the horror—and all of the reactions and emotions outlined in Dr. Goulston's 12 Phases Emotional Algorithm.

I tell it because, like many of the stories shared earlier in this book, my story illustrates and humanizes a lived experience with trauma and highlights the conditions that may lead to PTSD in an otherwise healthy and strong person.

And I tell it because, unknown to most at the time, I did develop PTSD, which eventually ended my career as I'd known it.

For years after the shooting, I effectively coped, mostly in positive and socially acceptable ways. I thought I was immune to PTSD—I'd been through many crises and disasters and was mentally tough. But toughness wasn't the antidote. Nor was busyness, though for many years it kept my symptoms at bay.

With the trauma not fully processed or resolved, and in the face of new threatening situations, my hypervigilance and isolation increased over the years, which led to depression and anxiety. For me, the shooting had shattered my sense of safety and security and unleashed a cascade of guilt, shame, and self-blame that haunted me in the aftermath. The hospital, which had previously felt safe and secure, was now a source of danger. PTSD lurked in plain sight. But it was only visible to me and my closest family members.

I could wholly function, and no one guessed that I had PTSD. At the time, adult-onset PTSD in civilians was not widely discussed or understood. Even though "PTSD" was a term commonly and flippantly used to describe the feelings someone might have following an upsetting situation or hardship, it was hardly an acceptable diagnosis for a professional, much less for the CEO. Its stigma was both real and felt.

Six years after the shooting and with a strong team in place, it was time for me to step aside, take a break, and get more intensive help. The organization deserved a healthy leader and I deserved to fully recover and heal. And after a lot of hard work and the help of experts in PTSD—using many of the therapies and techniques outlined in this book—I did just that. And now I'm in a position—with a new calling—to help other leaders and their organizations navigate severe crises and trauma.

Lastly, I tell this story because while PTSD is emerging as an expected and understandable consequence of COVID-19, it need not be an inevitable one.

PTSD NEED NOT BE INEVITABLE

As the pandemic rages on, action and intervention are necessary to ensure the well-being of our healthcare workforce. It's imperative that symptoms that arise in the face of this trauma are not ignored, downplayed, or dismissed and that the stigma of PTSD is not perpetuated because of a lack of knowledge or an unwillingness to learn. With good leadership (of ourselves and others), PTSD need not sneak up on anyone. And if it does develop, it can be treated and managed.

It is said that crisis makes the leader, but it also exposes poor ones. And a leader's actions, or inactions, greatly influence the ultimate impact of the trauma on people within an organization. Initially, and in the immediate aftermath of a trauma, leaders must focus on ensuring the safety of workers, unifying the workforce, and decreasing uncertainty to the greatest degree possible. And though leaders cannot always prevent or protect an organization from trauma, they can mitigate further harm to individuals and damage to the organization's culture by paying close attention to those conditions that make it hard for people to address their own physical and emotional well-being.

Leadership must be demonstrated from those most senior but need not only reside there. Leadership in the time of COVID-19 must be modeled at all levels, regardless of whether someone holds a title or rank or an official position. And each of us can model self-leadership. More than ever, authenticity, presence, compassion, equanimity, and empathy are needed from our leaders and for ourselves.

Throughout the COVID-19 crisis, there have been many examples of great leadership. The best leaders emphasize unity and connectedness. They are highly visible, convey messages directly (not just through a spokesperson), and express their own feelings of vulnerability in a genuine, balanced, and mature way. They take quick action when needed and are agile and responsive. They are responsible for themselves and for those in their charge. They communicate optimism, confidence, and resolve, and genuinely convey that "we're all in this together."

COMMUNICATION IS FUNDAMENTAL

Leaders always think they've communicated clearly and with enough information. Rarely is that true. Or they think they need to have all the answers or a perfectly written memo or email before communicating. In the absence of clear communication, a void is quickly created, and people don't generally fill voids with positive narratives, especially when they're in survival mode. People go into guessing mode and jump to conclusions, which many times veers far from the truth. During a crisis, good communication is fundamental to ensure accurate and timely information is provided, clear directives are given, and unnecessary uncertainty is minimized. To accomplish this, these are considered best practices:

- Leaders are highly visible and central to communication, even when there is a spokesperson or a call center in place.
- Be clear, remain consistent, and determine frequency—say how and when communication will occur and be clear about how people can get more information or have their questions answered.
- Be as simple and straightforward as possible: What is known— and what we're doing about it. What is not yet known—and what we're doing about it. Provide a timeline. Establish clear directives—what people need to do and when they need to do it.
- Communicate clearly about how decisions are being made or will be made. Remove any mystery. Don't forget to communicate the "why" in a decision.

- Use multiple modalities—FAQs, short videos, real-time town halls.

- Be willing to say, "I don't know," and follow it with, "but here's how I'm going to find out" and "this is when or how I'll get back to you."

- Be willing to admit mistakes and make course corrections. Much of what happens during a trauma is new territory. You may not have all the answers immediately and may make mistakes.

- Be willing to have difficult conversations. They rarely get easier when they are put off; avoidance usually makes the conflict worse and leads to distrust and lack of respect in leadership.

- If there are rumors or elephants in the room, address them. If no one brings them up, don't assume it's not an issue or a concern shared by many. Raise it yourself.

- Be upfront about any planned furloughs or pay cuts or layoffs. Be clear about how decisions will be made. And if there are not plans to reduce the workforce, make sure that's well known too!

- And, while persuasion and convincing are important elements in communicating a policy or a directive, shared learning is also an important goal and *listening* is indispensable to learning.

LISTENING IS INDISPENSABLE

When we're under great stress, it can be very difficult for any of us—and in particular leaders—to hear the angst, pain, resistance, and sometimes anger of others. Or to have it directed at us. But bearing witness to others' feelings is often what is most needed during and in the aftermath of a traumatic experience. Because in addition to the need for people to be heard and not placated, there is often important information underlying their concerns and worries. And there's a lot of wisdom found in the resistance that surfaces when we ask people to identify the pain points in an operation—and pause long enough to listen.

Organizations can face great peril in ignoring the insights of those on the front lines. It is this ability to be present, to really listen—and not just waiting for your turn to respond—that is crucial during trauma. A willingness to listen for things you don't want to hear is a vital leadership competency for solving complex and difficult problems that arise during trauma (and a useful best practice thereafter too).

SPECIFIC TRAUMA-INFORMED RESOURCES AND SUPPORT SERVICES ARE A MUST

Workers' fears and anxieties must be acknowledged as real and understandable. What people don't need to hear are pithy platitudes or superficial pep talks. They don't need to be told to "get over it" or "buck up." Their feelings are not unfounded or delusional. But these feelings also don't have to be unduly suppressed or denied, or hold the worker hostage. Nor do fear and anxiety always have to lead to chronic suffering or PTSD.

What workers need is a leader who models empathy for others' experiences and vulnerability of their own feelings. A leader who offers hope and acknowledges other people's feelings without fanning the flames of fear and worry. We often think that if we talk about stress or fear or anxiety that we'll dwell on it and make it worse. In my experience, the opposite is more likely—being able to express feelings and speak about fears in a psychologically safe environment leads to less isolation, which can be detrimental to well-being.

But leaders cannot, nor should they try to, do it alone or through solely utilizing internal resources. We can't stress enough the importance of getting expert help from the outside. The best organizations have established robust Employee Assistance Programs (EAP), peer-to-peer support groups, and access to one-on-one counseling. It's of utmost importance that the availability of psychological services is widely broadcast, and that staff members are encouraged to use them as needed. (Those who put up the bravest face may be the most at risk.)

History will indeed record the contributions of our healthcare professionals in response to the pandemic of 2020 and label them heroes. They've served under extreme duress and at enormous risk to themselves. We owe them a debt of gratitude, and they deserve our grace. And we are responsible for them. But time is of the essence, and the cost of inaction is great. We can and must save our healthcare workers from unnecessary suffering and disability. Let's answer the call to action and not let COVID-19 claim them as casualties or leave them behind after the battle with this pandemic is over.

ACKNOWLEDGMENTS

We'd like to thank our families and friends for their unending support and encouragement as we continue to pursue our lifelong commitment of making a difference in the lives of others.

A special thank you to our early readers of the manuscript, who provided honest feedback, insight, and suggestions: Steve Klasko, MD; Dave Logan; Lisa Majer, DO; Mary Ruppert, DO; and Lydia Vaias, MD.

Thank you to publisher Andrea Fleck-Nisbet, senior editor Amanda Bauch, and marketing director John Andrade of Harper Horizon, who have been enthusiastic and helpful partners in bringing this book to the world. Thank you for going above and beyond what we could have imagined.

And finally, we owe a debt of gratitude to our publicist, editor, and project manager extraordinaire, Dottie DeHart, and her amazing team, especially Eve Campbell and Megan Brendle. Without them, this book would not have been possible.

NOTES

Chapter 1: A Perfect Storm for Trauma

1. Amy Qin and Javier C. Hernández, "China Reports First Death from New Virus," *New York Times*, updated January 21, 2020, https://www.nytimes.com/2020/01/10/world/asia/china-virus-wuhan-death.html.

2. "Pelosi and Trump Reach Deal on a Relief Package," *New York Times*, March 13, 2020, https://www.nytimes.com/2020/03/13/world/coronavirus-news-live-updates.html.

3. Donald G. McNeil Jr., "The U.S. Now Leads the World in Confirmed Coronavirus Cases," *New York Times*, updated March 28, 2020, https://www.nytimes.com/2020/03/26/health/usa-coronavirus-cases.html.

4. Even Bush, "King County to Put 200-Bed Field Hospital on Shoreline Soccer Field Amid Coronavirus Outbreak," *Seattle Times*, March 18, 2020, https://www.seattletimes.com/seattle-news/health/king-county-to-put-200-bed-field-hospital-on-shoreline-soccer-field-amid-coronavirus-outbreak/; Jim Brunner, "A Look Inside the Army Field Hospital at CenturyLink Field, Designed to Help Medical Centers Swamped by Coronavirus Patients," *Seattle Times*, updated April 2, 2020, https://www.seattletimes.com/seattle-news/health/a-look-inside-the-army-field-hospital-at-centurylink-field-designed-to-help-medical-centers-swamped-by-coronavirus-patients/.

5. Meg Anderson, "Burials on New York Island Are Not New, But Increasing During Pandemic," NPR, April 10, 2020, https://www.npr

.org/sections/coronavirus-live-updates/2020/04/10/831875297/burials
-on-new-york-island-are-not-new-but-are-increasing-during-pandemic.
6. Antonio Noori Farzan et al., "Coronavirus Has Infected at Least
450,000 Health-Care Workers Worldwide, Report Says," *Washington Post*, June 3, 2020, https://www.washingtonpost.com/nation/2020
/06/03/coronavirus-live-updates-us/.
7. Christina Jewett, Melissa Bailey, and Danielle Renwick, "Exclusive:
Nearly 600 US Health Care Workers Have Died of COVID
-19," Kaiser Health News, June 8, 2020, https://khn.org/news
/exclusive-investigation-nearly-600-and-counting-us-health-workers
-have-died-of-covid-19/.

Chapter 2: The Frontline Experience

1. Jan Hoffman, "'I Can't Turn My Brain Off': PTSD and Burnout
Threaten Medical Workers," *New York Times*, May 16, 2020, https://
www.nytimes.com/2020/05/16/health/coronavirus-ptsd-medical
-workers.html.
2. Mental Health America: https://www.mhanational.org/find-support
-groups; NAMI (National Alliance on Mental Illness): https://www
.nami.org; National Center for PTSD: https://www.ptsd.va.gov
/gethelp/index.asp; PTSD Alliance: http://www.ptsdalliance.org
/help/; Sidran Institute Help Desk: https://www.sidran.org/help
-desk/; Suicide Prevention Lifeline: https://suicidepreventionlifeline
.org/.
3. Johnny Milano, "Infected But Feeling Fine: The Unwitting
Coronavirus Spreaders," *New York Times*, March 31, 2020, https://
www.nytimes.com/2020/03/31/health/coronavirus-asymptomatic
-transmission.html.
4. Dyani Lewis, "Mounting Evidence Suggests Coronavirus Is
Airborne—But Health Advice Has Not Caught Up," *Nature*, July 8,
2020, https://www.nature.com/articles/d41586-020-02058-1.
5. Paul P. Murphy and Theresa Waldrop, "Detroit Hospital Workers
Say People Are Dying in the ER Hallways Before Help Can Arrive,"
CNN.com, April 9, 2020, https://www.cnn.com/2020/04/09/us

/detroit-hospital-workers-sinai-grace-coronavirus/index.html; Jacki
Salo, "Disturbing Photos Show Body Bags Fill Hallways of Brooklyn
Hospital Amid Coronavirus," *New York Post*, April 5, 2020, https://
nypost.com/2020/04/05/disturbing-photos-show-body-bags-in
-hallways-of-nyc-hospital-amid-coronavirus/.

6. Jason Hill, "An ER Doctor's Diary of Three Brutal Weeks Fighting
COVID-19," BuzzFeed News, April 22, 2020, https://www
.buzzfeednews.com/article/jasonhill/coronavirus-covid
-19-er-doctor-diary-new-york-hospital.

7. Jillian Mock, "Psychological Trauma Is the Next Crisis for
Coronavirus Health Workers," *Scientific American*, June 1, 2020,
https://www.scientificamerican.com/article/psychological-trauma-is
-the-next-crisis-for-coronavirus-health-workers1/.

8. Lulu Garcia-Navarro, "What It's Like for Doctors on the Front Lines
of the Coronavirus Pandemic," NPR, March 29, 2020, https://www
.npr.org/2020/03/29/823438892/what-its-like-for-doctors-on-the-front
-lines-of-the-coronavirus-pandemic.

9. Emily Pierskalla, "I Want My Death to Make You Angry," Minnesota
Nurses Association (blog), April 2020, https://mnnurses.org/want-my
-death-make-you-angry/.

10. Arghavan Salles and Jessica Gold, "Health Care Workers Aren't
Just 'Heroes.' We're Also Scared and Exposed," Vox, April 2,
2020, https://www.vox.com/2020/4/2/21204402/coronavirus
-covid-19-doctors-nurses-health-care-workers.

11. Hoffman, "'I Can't Turn My Brain Off.'"

12. Hansi Lo Wang, "'I Hear the Agony': Coronavirus Crisis Takes Toll
on NYC's First Responders," NPR, April 23, 2020, https://www.npr
.org/2020/04/23/842011186/i-hear-the-agony-coronavirus-crisis-takes
-toll-on-nyc-s-first-responders.

13. Wang, "'I Hear the Agony.'"

14. Prateek Harne, "Doctor: I Am a Soldier in This Battle, and I Am
Scared," CNN, March 27, 2020, https://www.cnn.com/2020/03/27
/opinions/doctor-i-am-a-soldier-in-coronavirus-battle-and-i-am-scared
-harne/index.html.

15. Ann Cerniglia, "'What's It Like on the Front Lines? It's Hell,'" 4WWL, April 5, 2020, https://www.wwltv.com/article/news/health /coronavirus/whats-it-like-on-the-front-lines-its-hell/289-176e47e7 -47be-4cee-9705-489be57c3d93.

16. Olivia Carville et al., "What It's Like on the Front Lines of America's Battle with Coronavirus: A Surge of Virus Patients Pushes the U.S. Healthcare System to the Breaking Point," Bloomberg, March 27, 2020, https://www.bloomberg.com/news/features/2020-03-27/what -it-s-like-on-the-frontlines-of-america-s-battle-with-coronavirus.

17. Yuki Noguchi, "Trauma on the Pandemic's Front Line Leaves Health Workers Reeling," NPR, April 23, 2020, https://www.npr.org /sections/health-shots/2020/04/23/840986735/trauma-on -the-pandemics-front-line-leaves-health-workers-reeling.

18. Noguchi, "Trauma on the Pandemic's Front Line."

19. Eric Westervelt, "Can the U.S. Crowdsource Its Way Out of a Mask Shortage? No, But It Still Helps," NPR, March 25, 2020, https:// www.npr.org/2020/03/25/820795727/can-the-u-s-crowdsource-its -way-out-of-a-mask-shortage-no-but-it-still-helps.

20. Hill, "ER Doctor's Diary."

21. Jaclyn O'Halloran, "I'm a Nurse in a COVID-19 Unit. My Hospital's Leaders Scare Me More Than the Virus," STAT News, May 6, 2020, https://www.statnews.com/2020/05/06/nurse-frightened-hospital -administrators-more-than-covid-19/.

22. Carville et al., "What It's Like on the Front Lines."

23. Wang, "'I Hear the Agony.'"

24. Hill, "ER Doctor's Diary."

25. Corina Knoll, Ali Watkins, and Michael Rothfeld, "'I Couldn't Do Anything': The Virus and an E.R. Doctor's Suicide," *New York Times*, July 11, 2020, https://www.nytimes.com/2020/07/11/nyregion/lorna -breen-suicide-coronavirus.html.

26. Noguchi, "Trauma on the Pandemic's Front Line."

27. Wang, "'I Hear the Agony.'"

28. Jonathan Lloyd, "Doctor Moves into Tent in Garage to Protect His Family from Coronavirus," NBC Los Angeles, March 26, 2020,

https://www.nbclosangeles.com/news/coronavirus
/doctor-tent-garage-orange-county-irvine-california-covid-19
-coronavirus/2335884/.

29. Daniella Silva, "NYC Medical Residents Treating Coronavirus
Describe 'Living in a Nightmare,'" NBC News, April 16, 2020,
https://www.nbcnews.com/news/us-news/nyc-medical-residents
-treating-coronavirus-describe-living-nightmare-n1181386.

30. Ali Watkins et al., "Top E. R. Doctor Who Treated Virus Patients
Dies by Suicide," *New York Times*, updated April 29, 2020, https://
www.nytimes.com/2020/04/27/nyregion/new-york-city-doctor
-suicide-coronavirus.html.

31. Watkins et al., "Top E. R. Doctor."

32. Hoffman, "'I Can't Turn My Brain Off.'"

33. Elizabeth Findell, "In Texas, a Doctor Fights the Surge, and Gets
Covid-19; 'I Cry Every Day,'" *Wall Street Journal*, July 17, 2020,
https://www.wsj.com/articles/in-texas-a-doctor-fights-the-surge-and
-gets-covid-19-i-cry-every-day-11594891801.

34. Jenny Gross, "Nurses Who Battled Virus in New York Confront
Friends Back Home Who Say It's a Hoax," *New York Times*, July 7,
2020, https://www.nytimes.com/2020/07/07/us/coronavirus-nurses
.html.

35. "Health Equity Considerations and Racial and Ethnic Minority
Groups," CDC, July 24, 2020, https://www.cdc.gov
/coronavirus/2019-ncov/need-extra-precautions/racial-ethnic
-minorities.html.

36. Findell, "In Texas, a Doctor Fights the Surge."

37. Dan Diamond, "HHS Watchdog Vows Independence Amid Trump
Actions," Politico, May 26, 2020, https://www.politico.com
/news/2020/05/26/hhs-watchdog-vows-independence-amid
-trump-actions-282249.

38. Hannah Fry and Luke Money, "Orange County Public Health
Officer Resigns in Coronavirus Controversy," *LA Times*, June 9, 2020,
https://www.latimes.com/california/story/2020-06-09/orange-county
-public-health-officer-resigns-amid-controversy-over-face-coverings.

39. Katelyn Burns, "Governors Plead with Other States for More Health Care Workers to Fight Coronavirus," Vox, March 31, 2020, https://www.vox.com/policy-and-politics/2020/3/31/21201281/coronavirus-staffing-shortage-governors-health-care-workers-help.

40. Meghana Keshaven, "'We're Being Put at Risk Unnecessarily': Doctors Fume at Government Response to Coronavirus Pandemic," STAT, April 9, 2020, https://www.statnews.com/2020/04/09/doctors-fume-at-government-response-to-coronavirus-pandemic/.

41. Lena H. Sun and Josh Dawsey, "CDC Feels Pressure from Trump as Rift Grows Over Coronavirus Response," Washington Post, July 9, 2020, https://www.washingtonpost.com/health/trump-sidelines-public-health-advisers-in-growing-rift-over-coronavirus-response/2020/07/09/ad803218-c12a-11ea-9fdd-b7ac6b051dc8_story.html.

42. Brahma Chellaney, "Opinion: The World Health Organization Must Stop Covering Up China's Mistakes," MarketWatch, April 23, 2020, https://www.marketwatch.com/story/the-who-has-a-big-china-problem-2020-04-22.

43. "China Delayed Releasing Coronavirus Info, Frustrating WHO," CNBS, June 2, 2020, https://www.cnbc.com/2020/06/02/china-delayed-releasing-coronavirus-info-frustrating-who.html.

44. Sheryl Gay Stolberg, "Trump Administration Strips C.D.C. of Control of Coronavirus Data," New York Times, updated August 4, 2020, https://www.nytimes.com/2020/07/14/us/politics/trump-cdc-coronavirus.html.

45. Alice Miranda Ollstein, "Trump Halts Funding to World Health Organization," Politico, April 14, 2020, https://www.politico.com/news/2020/04/14/trump-world-health-organization-funding-186786.

46. Kathleen P. Harnett, et al., "Impact of the COVID-19 Pandemic on Emergency Department Visits—United States, January 1, 2019–May 30, 2020," Morbidity and Mortality Weekly Report 69 (2020): 699–704, http://dx.doi.org/10.15585/mmwr.mm6923e1.

47. Leila Fadel, "As Hospitals Lose Revenue, More than a Million Health Care Workers Lose Jobs," NPR, May 8, 2020, https://www.npr

.org/2020/05/08/852435761/as-hospitals-lose-revenue-thousands-of
-health-care-workers-face-furloughs-layoff.

48. Fadel, "As Hospitals Lose Revenue."

49. Ed Yong, "The Pandemic Experts Are Not Okay," *Atlantic*, July 7,
2020, https://www.theatlantic.com/health/archive/2020/07
/pandemic-experts-are-not-okay/613879/.

Chapter 3: The Aftershocks Are Coming

1. Lori Stahl, "Can Emergency Physician Stress Lead to Bigger
Problems?," ACEP Now, June 1, 2013, https://www.acepnow.com
/article/can-emergency-physician-stress-lead-bigger-problems/; Rick
Jervis, "'Death Is Our Greeter': Doctors, Nurses Struggle with
Mental Health as Coronavirus Cases Grow," *USA Today*, May 2,
2020, https://www.usatoday.com/story/news/nation/2020/05/03
/coronavirus-death-count-has-doctors-struggling-mental
-health/3063081001/.

2. Christine R. Stehman et al., "Burnout, Drop Out, Suicide: Physician
Loss in Emergency Medicine, Part 1," *Western Journal of Emergency
Medicine* 20, no. 3 (May 2019): 485–94, https://doi.org/10.5811
/westjem.2019.4.40970; Jervis, "'Death Is Our Greeter."

3. Catherine Burger, "What You Need to Know About Moral Injury,"
Minority Nurse, October 21, 2019, https://minoritynurse.com
/what-you-need-to-know-about-moral-injury/.

4. Jillian Mock, "Psychological Trauma Is the Next Crisis for
Coronavirus Health Workers," *Scientific American*, June 1, 2020,
https://www.scientificamerican.com/article/psychological-trauma-is
-the-next-crisis-for-coronavirus-health-workers1/.

5. Slew E. Chua et al., "Psychological Effects of the SARS Outbreak in
Hong Kong on High-Risk Health Care Workers," *Canadian Journal of
Psychiatry* 29, no. 6 (June 2004): 391–93, https://doi.org
/10.1177/070674370404900609; Rodrigo Pérez Ortega, "Health Care
Workers Seek to Flatten COVID-19's 'Second Curve'—Their Rising
Mental Anguish," Science, April 22, 2020, https://www.sciencemag

.org/news/2020/04/health-care-workers-seek-flatten-covid-19-s -second-curve-their-rising-mental-anguish.

6. Ping Wu et al, "The Psychological Impact of the SARS Epidemic on Hospital Employees in China: Exposure, Risk Perception, and Altruistic Acceptance of Risk," *Canadian Journal of Psychiatry* 54, no. 5 (May 2009): 302–11, https://doi.org/10.1177/070674370905400504.

7. Robert G. Maunder et al., "Long-Term Psychological and Occupational Effects of Providing Hospital Healthcare During SARS Outbreak," *Emerging Infectious Diseases* 12, no. 12 (December 2006): 1924–32, https://dx.doi.org/10.3201/eid1212.060584; Ortega, "Health Care Workers Seek to Flatten."

8. Neil Greenberg, Simon Wessely, and Til Wykes, "Potential Mental Health Consequences for Workers in the Ebola Regions of West Africa—A Lesson for All Challenging Environments," *International Journal of Mental Health* 24, no. 1 (February 2015): 1–3, https://doi .org/10.3109/09638237.2014.1000676; Shaili Jain, "Bracing for an Epidemic of PTSD Among COVID-19 Workers," *Psychology Today*, April 13, 2020, https://www.psychologytoday.com/us/blog/the -aftermath-trauma/202004/bracing-epidemic-ptsd-among-covid -19-workers.

9. Jianbo Lai et al., "Factors Associated with Mental Health Outcomes Among Health Care Workers Exposed to Coronavirus Disease 2019," *JAMA Network Open*, March 23, 2020, https://jamanetwork.com /journals/jamanetworkopen/fullarticle/2763229; Ortega, "Health Care Workers Seek to Flatten."

Chapter 5: The Road Back from Trauma

1. Tara E. Galovski, Sonya B. Norman, and Jessica Hamblen, "Cognitive Processing Therapy for PTSD," PTSD: National Center for PTSD, https://www.ptsd.va.gov/professional/treat/txessentials/cpt_for_ptsd _pro.asp.

ABOUT THE AUTHORS

MARK GOULSTON, MD, FAPA

Dr. Mark Goulston is a board-certified psychiatrist, Fellow of the American Psychiatric Association, former assistant clinical professor of psychiatry at UCLA NPI, and a former FBI and police hostage negotiation trainer. He is the creator of Theory Y Executive Coaching—which he provides to CEOs, presidents, founders, and entrepreneurs—and is a TEDx and international keynote speaker.

He is the creator and developer of Surgical Empathy, a process to help people recover and heal from PTSD, prevent suicide in teenagers and young adults, and help organizations overcome implicit bias.

Dr. Goulston is the author or principal author of seven prior books including *PTSD for Dummies*, *Get Out of Your Own Way: Overcoming Self-Defeating Behavior*, *Just Listen: Discover the Secret to Getting Through to Absolutely Anyone*, *Real Influence: Persuade Without Pushing and Gain Without Giving In*, and *Talking to Crazy: How to Deal with the Irrational and Impossible People in Your Life*. He hosts the *My Wakeup Call* podcast, where he speaks with thought leaders about their purpose in life and the wakeup calls that led them there. He also is the co-creator and moderator of the multihonored documentary *Stay Alive: An Intimate Conversation About Suicide Prevention*.

He appears frequently as a human psychology and behavior

subject-area expert across all media, including news outlets ABC, NBC, CBS, and BBC News, as well as CNN, *Today*, *Oprah*, the *New York Times*, the *Wall Street Journal*, *Forbes*, *Fortune*, *Harvard Business Review*, *Business Insider*, *Fast Company*, *Huffington Post*, and *Westwood One*. He was also featured in the PBS special "Just Listen."

DIANA HENDEL, PHARMD

Dr. Diana Hendel is an executive coach and leadership consultant, former hospital CEO, and author of *Responsible: A Memoir*, a riveting and deeply personal account of leading during and through the aftermath of a deadly workplace trauma.

As the CEO of Long Beach Memorial Medical Center and Miller Children's and Women's Hospital, Hendel led one of the largest acute care, trauma, and teaching hospital complexes on the West Coast. She has served in leadership roles in numerous community organizations and professional associations, including chair of the California Children's Hospital Association, executive committee member of the Hospital Association of Southern California, vice chair of the Southern California Leadership Council, chair of the Greater Long Beach Chamber of Commerce, board member of the California Society of Health-System Pharmacists, and leader-in-residence of the Ukleja Center for Ethical Leadership at California State University Long Beach.

She earned a BS in biological sciences from UC Irvine and a doctor of pharmacy degree from UC San Francisco. She has spoken about healthcare and leadership at regional and national conferences and at TEDx SoCal on the topic "Childhood Obesity: Small Steps, Big Change."